PREGNANCY GUIDE

THE ULTIMATE PREGNANCY GUIDE PACKAGE

SARAH KATE BUTTERSON

ISBN: 9781720284338

TABLE OF CONTENTS

CHAPTER ONE 4

DISCOVER HOW TO MAXIMIZE YOUR CHANCES OF GETTING PREGNANT 4

BRIEF INTRODUCTION TO CONCEPTION...................................5

PREPARATION TO INCREASE THE CHANCES OF CONCEPTION 8

MEASURING AND PLANNING FERTILITY 19

CHAPTER TWO...36

GETTING ALL THE RIGHT FOOD AND NUTRITION DURING A PREGNANCY ...36

INTRODUCTION TO CALORIES: EATING FOR TWO 38

NUTRIENTS THAT PLAY A KEY ROLE IN PREGNANCY.....................43

FOOD AND SUBSTANCES WORTH AVOIDING DURING PREGNANCY 59

FOOD SAFETY DURING PREGNANCY 63

FINAL WORDS ON EATING RIGHT DURING PREGNANCY...................68

CHAPTER THREE 70

ABSOLUTELY EVERYTHING YOU NEED TO KNOW ABOUT LABOR AND DELIVERY 70

IDENTIFYING THE SIGNS AND SYMPTOMS OF PRE-LABOR........................72

STARTING TO GO INTO LABOR: WHAT YOU SHOULD DO? AND HOW TO HANDLE IT!...80

FACING BOTH LABOR AND DELIVERY 85

FINAL WORDS ON LABOR AND DELIVERY...............................98

CHAPTER FOUR...101

EVERYTHING YOU NEED TO KNOW ABOUT GETTING STARTED WITH

PRENATAL WORKOUTS 101

INTRODUCTION TO PRENATAL WORKOUTS 102

COMPLETE PREPARATION FOR PRENATAL WORKOUTS.............107

GETTING STARTED WITH EXERCISE 116

TYPES OF PRENATAL WORKOUTS..120

STARTING YOUR OWN WORKOUTS, TODAY! 133

CHAPTER FIVE...135

ABSOLUTELY EVERYTHING THAT YOU MUST HAVE FOR AN UPCOMING BABY BOY OR GIRL 135

"WHEN SHOULD I START THE PREPARATION?" 137

ABSOLUTE ESSENTIALS FOR A NEW ARRIVAL 139

MUCH NEEDED EXTRAS FOR A NEWBORN 158

GETTING EVERYTHING THAT YOUR CHILD NEEDS READY 165

CHAPTER SIX..168

WORKING YOUR WAY BACK TO TERRIFIC SHAPE AFTER A PREGNANCY....168

WEIGHT GAIN AND PREGNANCY...170

EVERYTHING YOU NEED TO KNOW ABOUT CALORIES 173

FIRMLY RESOLVING TO LOSE WEIGHT AFTER PREGNANCY 177

BEFORE YOU BEGIN ANY WEIGHT LOSS EFFORT... 180

STARTING TO TRIM DOWN RIGHT AFTER PREGNANCY.............185

FINDING WAYS TO FIT IN A WORKOUT ROUTINE 191

GRADUALLY UPPING THE ANTE OF YOUR WEIGHT LOSS 195

GETTING IN SHAPE AND STAYING IN SHAPE.............................201

CHAPTER ONE

Discover How to Maximize Your Chances of Getting Pregnant

Wanting to get pregnant is simply the first step in a very long road that lies before you. For some, things fall into place rather simply, especially the pregnancy itself. Actually, some people have trouble not getting pregnant

But for many others, they quickly discover that getting pregnant may not be as simple as they first imagined.

Depending on a diversity of factors, you may find that it is slightly difficult, or even close to impossible, to get pregnant. While, granted, on occasion the problem is very serious, most times it is something that can be dealt with – and pretty simply at that.

All that you need is to approach it in the right manner, so that your probabilities of getting pregnant are really maximized, and this means developing an understanding of pregnancy itself, and dealing with the factors that are behind it.

Over this guide, we are going to go through a complete discovery process of many various things that you can do to help increase your chances and probabilities of getting pregnant.

By giving you all the knowledge, you shouldn't only have a better understanding of pregnancy itself, but you also must be able to get out there and start doing something about getting pregnant – almost instantly!

Before we get started, it would likely be a good idea to go over a fast recap of what pregnancy really entails. Sure, it's the kind of stuff that you probably learnt in a sex education or biology classroom back when you were a child, but just consider this a 'refresher' course that is going to set the stage for learning how to get pregnant.

Are you ready to get started?

Brief Introduction to Conception

Naturally, you know by now that pregnancy is the process by which women carry children to term, and then deliver them. Yes, that's right, children are born not brought over by storks during the night.

But, seeing as the central point of this entire guide is about how to actually get pregnant, what we are interested in is what actually goes on to cause pregnancy, and this is, as you may have estimated, known as 'conception'. Or, in other words: Fertilization.

Essentially, for human beings like us, fertilization is the union of an egg and a sperm. As you can well expect, the females provide the eggs, and the males provide the sperm, and the union takes place within the female womb.

And yes, sex is exactly the process by which the sperm is inserted into the female body, before it journey's to the uterus and causes conception.

Although all of this is totally basic stuff, you might have guessed by now that there is truly a lot more to conception than simply this. After all, if it was just a question of having sex, then there'd be no issue at all. In fact, there are many problems involved with this process.

Firstly, any ejaculated sperm need to actually make it to the uterus, and not all will most of the time. But far more importantly, even once sperm do make it that far, there really needs to be an egg there for fertilization to happen.

That is one of the key prerequisites for any pregnancy to happen: A woman needs to actually be at a stage of her menstrual cycle where an egg has been released and is prepared for fertilization. Otherwise, it easily cannot happen.

On top of that, at specific points, the probabilities of fertilization are vastly maximized, meaning that your chances of getting pregnant would be great at certain times.

Further to this, there are other factors to. For example, even the moment that a woman is ovulation, and sperm does get where they should be, that does not necessarily mean that fertilization is going to happen.

Sometimes, for a variety of reasons, it doesn't. Without getting too medical, it would be great if you think of it this way: For some reasons, the sperm might not be able to get into the egg in order to form the 'union' that it needs to.

End of the day, you now have a rough sufficient idea of what conception entails.

By this point, you possibly even have pinpointed at least one of the topics that is going to form a big portion of what this guide is concerning. Yes, that's right: Finding out once the best point in time for fertilization to occur.

Soon enough, we'll get to that, but currently, there is some starting points that ought to help maximize your chances of getting pregnant. Really, they're the very first port of call that you should be considering, and so we should absolutely deal with them right now!

Preparation to Increase the Chances of Conception

Knowing as you currently do (and probably already did!) that both men and women have roles to play in a successful pregnancy, it makes sense that there are specific items in terms of preparation that each ought to undertake.

Bear in mind that these are, as mentioned, the type of things that should be done as fast as possible.

So, as soon as you are done with this section, you should be willing to begin at least making an effort to get some of them done. Sure, you could wait until you are done reading this guide, but don't forget!

Some of what we are about to discuss will be based on the factors that play a role in conception. Admittedly, we haven't really discussed these in depth, but they are the kind of thing that you will become very accustomed to as we go along.

Plus, to discuss them in ton of detail would mean getting very technical, and unless you want a crash course in biology, it is best that we steer clear of that for now.

Anyway, first, let's look at the preparation that women must undertake to initially raise their chances of conception.

Preparation for Women

Being a woman, the role that's played in pregnancy is a very major one, unnecessary to say. In conception, that role is no less important, as it is the woman's primary mission to supply the egg for fertilization.

As we explore the steps that a woman could, and should, take in order to increase their chances to get pregnant, you will notice that a lot of it does tie in to what we discussed earlier regarding fertility.

Don't worry if your grasp on fertility is not entirely firm yet – we will be covering it in greater depth later.

Now, here is some of the steps that you should be starting to carry out:

1. Stop All Forms of Birth Control

Sure, it does not take a rocket scientist to discover that the most important thing that you need to do is to stop any birth control measures that you may be on. But depending on the type of birth control that you have been taking, you might find that there are other factors that need consideration.

For example, once an intra-uterine device (IUD) or 'the pill' mostly have no long- standing consequences, other birth control forms, like Depo-Provera, the birth control injection, may anything from 9 months to a year before they stop being effective.

Plan accordingly, because if you are on some form of birth control that requires you to cease well in advance, well, you should absolutely stop it right now.

Consult a doctor or pharmacist if you need any furthermore a piece of advice regarding the specific type of birth control that you are on. And don't worry – if you are just on the pill, it isn't going to affect your chances and probabilities of getting pregnant once you stop.

While you've dealt with your birth control, you have taken the first firm step toward getting pregnant.

2. Try to Reduce Stress

Although the jury is still out regarding the specific impact of stress on fertility, and hence, the chances of getting pregnant, numerous studies have shown that a link of sorts does exist. Anyway, being stress free is generally a great idea all in all.

Essentially, if you can, try to both avoid stressful situations as much as possible, and relax yourself in those inevitable times when you will inevitably get stressed.

Some techniques, like meditation, massages, and the like are absolutely great ways to get started. Of course, easily taking deep breaths and trying to calm yourself is just as good, provided you are the sort of person for whom that suffices.

Assuming that for any reason, you are constantly faced with potentially stressful situations, you might want to find more fixed outlets by which you can relieve your stress.

End of the day, being stress free is absolutely something that could help you to get pregnant, so try hard!

3.   Quit Smoking

Despite the fact that it is easier said than done, quitting smoking is the best thing that you could do.

For a woman, the risks that smoking presents in terms of pregnancy are diversified, and fearsome. Firstly, not solely does it affect a woman's general fertility, but smoking has also been shown to dramatically maximize the chances of miscarriages occurring. However the risks don't just stop there. In fact, it gets worse.

Babies of smokers end up bearing the brunt of the effects, and tend to weigh less on birth. As well, there is a big risk of them being born prematurely, which in itself, can carry many other risks along with it.

Studies have also gone to show that these children always end up suffering from numerous effects that are tied in with second hand smoke. Some of these effects include things such as asthma, bronchitis, and even, in some bad cases, cancer.

All of these risks truly do paint a pretty grim picture for smokers. And, even though they are just 'risks', and hardly set in stone, the question that you must be asking yourself is: Why risk it? So, if you are able to, start to try to quit smoking NOW!

Today, there are many aids that can help you do so, from nicotine patches, right on to inhalers, and many other things. Most doctors would readily be able to support you with any further advice.

3. Ensure that You Are a Healthy Weight

Some imagine that being a 'healthy' weight means that they need to lose weight. This is not true in the slightest. In fact, it's just as bad being underweight as it is overweight, so don't simply go on a diet for no reason!

Data has showed that women who are their ideal weight get pregnant more easily than their fellows who are either under, or over, weight.

If you need to lose weight, then you might want to do so through exercise combined with a diet, rather than just a diet alone. Overall, the benefits of exercising are good, and so you must take full advantage of them!

On the other hand, if you need to gain a little bit of weight, well, indulge a little in terms of food!

Each of these four steps that we have discussed must be taken into account and implemented as fast as you can. Of course, if you are a man then this does not apply, at least not in the way that we have outlined. However there are some things that do…

Preparation for Men

From what you previously know about fertilization, the role of the man is to provide sperm that are strong enough to reach and penetrate the female's egg.

With this in mind, it mustn't be too much of a leap to realize that any and all preparation that you undertake needs to be centered on that core idea: Ensuring that your sperm is of enough strength to do his job.

Of course it isn't that easy. No matter what, a single sperm's chances of success are slim, to say the least. That's why, in a single ejaculation, countless sperm are unleashed at once. And the exact number of these sperm varies from person to person.

Thus, apart from just strengthening your sperm, maximizing the number that is unleashed would be equally beneficial to your opportunities. This 'number' is referred to as the sperm count. Let's look at what you must be starting to do:

1.   Quit Smoking

Let's discuss smoking a little. Now, you previously know how it affects women, so there is no need to go over that again, however there are other affects that should worry men.

Particularly, this revolves around the simple fact that smoking has been proven to cause reduced sperm counts.

Moreover, even secondhand smoke from a man can cause a woman to face all the effects of smoking itself, which simply continues to compound the situation. Bear in mind that this works vice versa too, i.e. secondhand smoke from a woman can cause a man to have a lower sperm count.

But, the great news is that if you do manage to kick that smoking habit, you can expect your sperm count to raise dramatically. In some cases, this rise has even been recorded to be up to 800%, which is, as you can probably appreciate, nothing less than astounding. So quit smoking, right now!

2.   Get Sufficient Vitamins and Minerals

Depending on how your diet is balanced, you may or may not have problems in this regard. In particular, you should be watching your Vitamin E and C intake, as well as whether or not you are getting sufficient zinc.

All of these nutrients have been shown to help rise the well being and mobility of your sperm, strengthening them, and also maximizing the chances that they will manage to fertilize an egg.

Assuming you are not able to change your diet to get sufficient of these vitamins and minerals, then you must perhaps consider taking supplements that could help you achieve the same desired affect. So long as you're getting the nutrients somehow, you should be fine.

3.   Dodge Toxins, and Stop Recreational Drug Use

Overall, toxins and drugs have a very adverse affect on sperm in men, both in terms of the sperm count, and their power. Because of this, you must definitely dodge toxins as much as possible, and stop taking any recreational drugs that you might sometimes indulge in.

Some recreational drugs even end up decreasing the male sex drive, which could be a very bad thing indeed, mostly if you are already facing issues conceiving.

As far as toxins go though, what you have to be worried about are things such as heavy metals, pesticides, and other chemicals. Constant exposure to such things may cause other problems too.

Remember this, and try, as much as humanly possible, to decrease your exposure to both these things.

4.   Try to Avoid High Temperatures

Once exposed to high temperatures, you could very well find that your sperm production is negatively affected as studies have proven.

A few points of interest in this regard would be to, first and foremost, wear loose underwear that does not trap hot air. Apart from that though, you must also avoid long hot baths, saunas, and other such things. Anything that could expose you to high temperatures must be avoided.

5.   Exercise in Moderation

In essence, the amount of exercise that you must be aiming for is something along the lines of 'enough, but not too much'. Don't overdo it.

Once getting some exercise can be helpful to your sexual health, going to extremes could truly reduce your sperm count. This is due to the fact that over- exercising actually decreases the amount of testosterone in your body – and that will result in a lower sperm count.

Basically, keep it in moderation, and you must be able to enjoy the benefits of exercising, without its potential ill effects.

Try to put these preparatory efforts into action as soon as possible. As you have noticed, some of them will need working on, however at the end of the day, the rewards nature worth the effort that you put in.

Naturally, a joint effort is the best kind, and both the man and woman in a partnership must be doing their part to guarantee that the best chances of a pregnancy can be achieved.

Having gone over this first preparation, let's move on to something that is at the core of how to get pregnant, and really, an extension of the fertilization concepts that we have been discussing earlier.

Measuring and Planning Fertility

Already, you know the basics of fertility and how it works. Just to recap and reassert what you know though, here is the lowdown:

Every month, an egg is, invariably, released, and this is called ovulation. As the egg travels down the fallopian tube, it's then the perfect time for fertilization to happen. But, this is, unfortunately, not a process that is very easily timed.

Although the standard rule of thumb is that women have a 28 day cycle, the truth is that for many women, this does tend to vary from month to other. Furthermore, even for those that do have a regular-as-clockwork 28 day cycle, the exact time when the egg is ideally placed for fertilization can still vary.

As you might have supposed, this makes it tough to measure and plan for the 'most fertile' moment, and so you are going to have to rely on some other methods rather than merely counting days.

First though, you must know roughly how your cycle works in the first place.

Charting and Recording Ovulation Cycles

Okay, although this is not the most trustworthy way of determining when you are most fertile, it is still a great starting point.

Generally, if you have a regular 28-day cycle, your ovulation is going to begin 14 days after the day your last period began. That said, this can vary by as much as a few days, and is bound to vary more in women who do not have a regular 28 day cycle.

In such cases, the best way is to keep track of how long your cycles normally are. Then, pick the shortest one and subtract 18 from the number of days that it lasted. When the next period begins, add this amount of days and track that point in time. For a week following that tracked point, you must be at your most fertile.

Sure, this is only an approximation, however the reason that it is such a great starting point is that it should help you get a rough idea of the period when you should start to try to notice, or measure, some of the other factors that we are going to be talking about now.

Measuring Basal Body Temperature

Simply put, basal body temperature is a temperature taken while the body is at rest. That means it should be taken immediately after you wake up, and before you do any sort of physical activity.

To do so, you will need more than just a regular thermometer. Specialized basal thermometers are commonly sold, and these are going to be far more precise than the regular set – which is what you need because the temperature difference that you are tracking is less than a degree.

Basically the theory is this – during ovulation, a woman's basal body temperature rises anything from 0.3 to 0.8 degrees Fahrenheit.

Thus, by keeping track of the basal body temperature, you can pinpoint the exact point at which ovulation happen.

In order for this to be most effective, you need to keep track of your basal body temperature over the span of two or more periods. Start recording your basal body temperature instantly after you get a period, and then continue to do so throughout.

Having a calendar, or chart, to keep track of the temperature on a daily basis is maybe going to be of great help.

Once you have noticed the increase, and noted it, over the span of a few periods, you must be able to then predict when your ovulation is going to happen. After that, simply look to the 2 or 3 days prior to that temperature increase, and mark these down as your most fertile days!

Simple isn't it?

Just remember that you will want to regularly record your basal body temperature at the same time every day, and you will need at very least three hours of sleep before you take a recording.

All in all, this method of measurement is much more effective than simply 'guessing', but there are other telltale signs that could also help you out even further…

Keeping an Eye Out for Cervical Mucus

Chances are, you have already noticed cervical mucus, even if you don't know what it is. At different times, you most likely have noticed that your underwear was wet.

In reality, this dampness is caused by cervical mucus, which will alter and be discharged to help sperm move towards the egg when you're most fertile. Keep this in mind because it means that once you notice it – that is your most fertile point.

What you are looking for is cervical mucus that strongly resembles raw egg whites. At the beginning, when you first notice cervical mucus discharges, it will perhaps be thicker, and creamier in color.

Eventually though, it will change, and spotting this change is what you need to accomplish.

By regularly checking your cervical fluid, either every day, or better yet, any time you visit the bathroom, you could record what you notice in a chart – possibly even the same one that you use to record basal temperatures.

Following this, you should be able to further regularly pinpoint your most fertile point, and use this information to your advantage.

Keep in mind though, some feminine hygiene products, like douches, can actually alter your cervical fluid, which will make it harder (or even impossible!) for you to notice any changes occurring in them.

Also, any and all judgment of cervical fluid is bound to be fully subjective, thus it may take some time before you can actually start to know for certain that you are noticing the right thing.

Coupled with the changes that you notice in your basal temperature though, you should be able to, by this point, somewhat accurately pinpoint the times at which you are most fertile.

Alternative Measures for Fertility Prediction

If, after everything we have covered, you find that you still have problems predicting exactly when you are most fertile, don't despair. Today, there are a number of other alternatives that you can follow, but none is as popular as the ovulation predictor kits that are most often used.

In theory, these kits work on easy logic: Before ovulation, the production of certain hormones rises within a woman's body. By testing for the presence of these hormones, it's really possible to identify the time of ovulation, or even the period leading up to it.

Almost all over-the-counter prediction kits work in roughly the same way, and include testing urine samples for hints of increased hormone production.

But, it is highly recommended that you take a look at the instructions of the specific type of predictor kit that you are using, thus that you are able to get accurate results. Some of these kits can be quite expensive too, so if you are on a limited budget, you would probably be better off sticking with the more traditional methods.

As accurate as the results from such kits can be though, there is one risk that many individuals actually end up falling afoul of – and that is that they end up trying to 'time' sex so precisely that they really end up missing the most fertile point.

Don't make this error, and you should find that prediction kits are a true asset to have on your side.

Well, now that you know how to predict the most fertile point, you are almost there in terms of knowing the best ways to rise your chances and probabilities of a pregnancy. But before we are quite done, you must know how to actually take advantage of this most fertile point...

Taking Full Advantage of Fertility

Being able to measure and predict, and therefore plan for, precisely when you are going to be most fertile is great – but taking advantage of that knowledge is very much indispensable if you want to get pregnant.

Although you may think that this is the simple part, don't be fooled into a false sense of security.

While it's true that sex is, basically, the method by which you take advantage of fertility, the truth is that sometimes it does not suffice. Sometimes, there needs to be other measures taken in tandem, to further maximize your chances.

Here and now, we are going to walk you through some of the steps that you must be taking in order to make the most of all the planning that you have done.

Think of these steps as the sort of things that could prove to tip the scale of opportunity in your favor. Assuming you have tried before, and failed, to get pregnant, then some of these steps could make all the difference in your efforts.

Sexual Related Tips to Improve the Chances of Conception

Well, as you already realize, sex is at the very core of whether or not you end up getting pregnant. Remember, you should know that there are many things you should also know about sex to ensure that you get the best results.

None of these tips are really very out of the ordinary, but they will each increase your chances a little, and in tandem, work together to help you to get pregnant.

Take a glance through the following:

1.   Try to Have Sex Regularly

During the fertile period, you must be having sex as regularly as possible. In fact, there is no harm with having sex regularly throughout the year, and it will surely be beneficial in terms of your efforts to get pregnant.

Despite the fact that you should have pinpointed the most fertile part of your cycle, trying to just hit that one target alone is, really, ill advised.

After all, if you happen to be off by even a little bit, you will end up both being too late or too early, so, all your efforts will amount to nothing.

On the other hand, if you are having sex regularly over that period, your chances of hitting the target are actually improved. At very least you must come close multiple times, and this would up the possibility that you will conceive.

In short: There is no such thing as too much sex.

The reason that many couples who are trying to conceive truly end up having less sex than they should is the folktale that it will lower a man's sperm count if he has too much sex.

This is, as mentioned, just a folktale. In fact, having regular sex isn't going to affect any man's sperm count much, unless he has some preexisting condition that makes it so. If this is the case, then you must be consulting a doctor.

Normally, the reduction in sperm count due to regular sex is so minute that it's negligible.

Essentially, having sex regularly is absolutely the way to go.

2.   Stay off Artificial Lubricants

Many individuals don't know this yet, however artificial lubricants have been found to be toxic to sperm, and can absolutely hinder your chances of getting pregnant.

Normally, the existing acidic secretions in the vagina do kill off sperm naturally, but, during the fertile period, the cervical mucus that's featured helps to protect the sperm.

By using artificial lubricants, you are basically going to be 'blocking' the sperm from reaching the safety of the cervical mucus, so, they are going to end up dying in the acidic secretions instead.

Bottom line: As far as possible, stay off any artificial lubricants.

If you actually do need some form of lubrication, then try using warm water, which will not interfere with the sperm's ability to reach the cervical mucus. Or, as a final resort, just using a very small amount of KY jelly mixed with water should not have too big an adverse effect. Still, the best way is definitely to go all natural!

3.   Choosing the Right Position

Don't get confused – you can get pregnant if you have sex in any position that you like, but some positions have been shown to maximize your chances slightly – and that could make all the difference.

In a nutshell, positions that require the sperm to defy gravity and swim 'upstream, so to speak, like sitting, standing, or with the woman on top, are definitely the sort of thing that you must avoid.

On the other hand, the simplicity of the missionary position is absolutely something that helps out.

All in all, if you're having issues conceiving, and you do often use some of the aforementioned 'gravity defying' positions, then maybe you could try switching back to plain ol' missionary for a while.

4.   Don't Use a Douche after Sex

Honestly, this really is just common sense, but using a douche after sex is going to negatively influence your chances.

Douching will inevitably alter the pH levels of the vagina,so as you already know, could end up killing sperm. Moreover, any cervical mucus might be flushed out, which is what helps sperm to travel to the uterus.

End of the day: Don't douche!

5.   Keep Sex Fun

Now, one of the key things that many individuals often end up forgetting in their quest to get pregnant is to simply have fun. Sex is meant to be fun, and you must definitely try to keep it that way.

If you get too stressed and serious or tense about getting pregnant, then you are going to end up finding that sex is less fun, and more of a chore.

As a result, you are also perhaps going to end up having less sex overall than you otherwise would, which is going to be detrimental to your chances and probability of getting pregnant. Also, as you know from way earlier, stress could also lower your chances further.

Try new things, and be sure to take into consideration the needs of your partner, so that both of you end up having a good time.

Should you be able to keep sex fun, and carry it out as often as possible, you will find that you will probably have little or no problem getting pregnant!

All of these sexual related tips form the core of your efforts to get pregnant. And, as promised, none of them are especially tough to carry out, are they?

Of course, apart from sexual related tips, there are a few other things that can also help to rise your conception chances, and before we leave you to your own devices, how about we skim through some of these…

Other Tips and Advice to Help Get Pregnant

Already, we have covered a lot of methods that should help increase your chances of getting pregnant. Now, we are in the final lap, and it's time that we go over a few last efforts that must be undertaken.

Keep in mind that these are no less important than anything else that we have discussed so far!

Some of these tips are the sort of thing that we have already discussed, however must definitely be reiterated, as you will see:

1.   Keep Healthy

On the whole, keeping healthy, both through sport and a balanced diet, could help your efforts to get pregnant. And, even more than that, this healthy lifestyle will also help you and your baby during the pregnancy itself.

Try to cut out any caffeine from your diet as much as possible.

2.   Cut Out Smoking, Recreational Drugs, and Alcohol

Already, we have discussed why smoking and recreational drugs are bad, and it must come as no surprise to you that alcohol is just as bad. Both of these habits can affect your chances of getting pregnant, and could also affect the health and well being of your baby if you do get pregnant.

Staying away from all these substances is something that you must do!

3.   Take Folic Acid

Folic acid, or rather, Vitamin B-9, is a vitamin that is known to help pregnancy, and play a role in a baby's development. Although it is not directly linked to conception, it's something that you must be thinking of doing, at very least.

Armed with these final tips, you are ready to go out there and start trying to get pregnant. Just a few words of advice, and we will let you do just that!

Final Words: "If All Else Fails…"

Over this guide, we have covered practically everything that you need to know about getting pregnant. With the knowledge that you have now, you must be able to dramatically improve your chances of doing so.

But, sometimes that just is not enough. Sometimes, there are genetic and medical issues at work that even all of what you now know can not help you with.

In these cases, you will have no choice but to consult a doctor or fertility expert, and get some medical advices, and possibly, drugs, which could help your efforts. Don't surrender hope though, and certainly, don't resort to that until you have tried what we have taught you.

Despite the fact that these measures may not be effective in some cases, in most cases they really are, as many people who have trouble conceiving really just are not going about things in the most effective manner.

Already, you must have possibly seen some areas in which you could improve, so go out there and get to it!

CHAPTER TWO

Getting All the Right Food and Nutrition during a Pregnancy

Without a doubt, you probably previously realize that getting the right sort of nutrition is important during your pregnancy. After all – you are now going to be having another living being relying on you to obtain all of his or her nutrition needs as well, which makes it vital that you are able to give your child what he or she requires.

But, this does not mean that you should just wait until you conceive to start eating the right types of foods. Chances are, you will only discover that you have conceived anything from a day or two right up to a week after you actually have.

Due to this, it's very much advisable that you start eating right from the very minute that you actually think about having a baby.

Contrary to popular belief, getting the right food and nutrition does not have to be about eating savourless and bland meals. In fact, it's completely possible to have healthy meals that are very tasty too.

Over this guide, we are going to be looking at the different nutrients that you must definitely be consuming.

If you know a bit about nutrition already, some of these should make sense to you. Others may take a little explaining before you can grasp their significance, but it's important that you do.

By knowing the nutrients that you, and your baby, need, you will be better able to understand why it's so vital that you obtain them somehow.

Before we begin jumping straight into the nutrients though, there are is one other area in particular that we are going to deal with: Calories. Don't worry if you are not exactly an expert on calories, however chances are if you have ever gone on a diet before, you are at least somewhat familiar with them.

Anyway, we will give you the whole picture regarding calories and how they relate to your pregnancy shortly.

For now, just keep in mind: What you should want to be learning from this guide is how to eat well, so that your baby ends up benefiting from having all the necessary nutrients for his or her growth.

Needless to say, this must be more than enough motivation for you to want to really get your teeth into what this guide has to offer, so let's go ahead and kick things off on that note.

Introduction to Calories: Eating for Two

A 'calorie' is a word that invariably ends up getting tied in with exercise, dieting and losing weight in general.

Thus, it should not surprise you too much that this tie in also applies when eating during pregnancy, though in a slightly different way. Generally, this is due to the fact that you aren't really concerned about losing weight.

To start off with, let's take a look at calories. On a basic level, calories are a measure of energy, so when this is applied to food, they signify the amount of energy you are able to get out of a certain food type.

Simple enough right?

Surely, different types of foods give different amount of energy. For example, fat provides more energy per gram than carbohydrates or proteins. Although this is an important distinction for weight loss, it's less so for our purposes.

During a pregnancy, because you are now eating for both you and your child, it makes sense that you would need more energy, both for yourself, and for the child. However, this does not mean that your food intake must double, and that's why the phrase 'eating for two' really isn not very accurate.

Yes, you're eating for two, but no, you aren not going to be eating double the calories.

Normally, your calorie intake must only rise by about 15%, or, in other words, roughly 300 calories or so. To put this into perspective, it's about the equivalent of 3 cups of non-fat milk.

Does not sound like much does it – but that is the key point here. However yes, you can eat more if you want to, you really don't have to, and 300 calories is more than enough to support both you and your child's needs.

But, for those 300 calories to be enough, you need to make them count.

Keeping this in mind, there are 2 general ways in which people rise their calorie count:

1.   Eating a lot of junk food or high-calorie products

2.   Eating more nutritious food that fills up the calories

Essentially, if you follow the first path, you will need to consume more calories just so that you end up filling up enough nutrients for your child. Of course, if you are ensuring that the extra 300 calories that you are taking on already does just that, then you will end up consuming less calories overall.

End of the day, the latter path is very much the desired one, as not just is it healthier, but it will also mean that you don't put on too much undesirable weight. Some weight gain during pregnancy is natural – however you can ensure that you are not going to have to spend months trying to lose all of it just by eating right!

Speaking of which, how about we quickly address some of the misconceptions about weight gain and eating during pregnancy…

Brief Glance at Weight Gained During Pregnancy

Because weight gain is inexplicably connected to calories, it makes sense that we discuss this just to get it out of the way. From the start though, you must know: Most of the weight that you gain during pregnancy isn't fat, and thus not connected to calories at all.

Many women make one simple error though: They figure that since a baby only weighs about 7.5 pounds, they should not be gaining much more than that. This is completely false, and in fact, it's really normal to gain as much as 25 to 35 pounds, or more.

End of the day, the exact amount of weight gained varies depending on a lot of factors.

Of course, if you are carrying twins, or triplets, you would expect to gain more, but for the standard pregnancy, this is how the weight gained generally breaks down:

First, there is the baby's weight that ends up being roughly 7.5 pounds. Apart from that though, there are other items, like extra stored proteins and fats, extra blood, and other extra body fluids that account for about 15 pounds more.

Further to that, there are also some other changes going on in your body, like breast enlargement, womb enlargement, placenta, and amniotic fluid surrounding the baby, that make up the rest of the weight.

As you can see, all in all, that is far more than the weight of your baby alone.

Knowing this should equip you with one key piece of information, and that just because you are gaining weight, it does not mean that you should be watching your calorie intake more carefully. Sure, keep it to 300 calories or so extra, but don not cut it down from that amount at the expense of crucial nutrients.

Everything that your baby needs is in the nutrients, and so cutting back on that will adversely impact your baby's health and development.

Having gone over calories, and also touched on weight gain, it is time we look past those things, and get right down to the meat of this guide. And yes, that means discussing nutrients.

Nutrients That Play a Key Role in Pregnancy

Now that we are getting down to the nutrients themselves, you can expect to be getting a lot of information that's going to directly relate to what you eat. Long story short, every piece of food you eat is perhaps made up of multiple components…

Unnecessary to say, you could classify 'better' food as those types of food that have many various nutrients packed into them. Similarly, the 'not-so-good' food would be more of the set that have little or no nutrients to speak of, and are just compromised of mostly carbohydrates or fat.

On the other side of the spectrum, there'd be the 'bad' food, and we will get to an explanation of this later on.

For now, we are interested in the nutrients themselves, so let's get started by looking at some of the more mutual components that are going to play a role in your pregnancy.

Protein

Without getting very technical, it would be best for us to think of proteins as 'building blocks', so to speak. Call them what you will, there are basically about 20 various types of proteins, or rather, 'amino acids', as the proper term is.

Protein has various roles, but not the least of which is in the area of cell production. In short, proteins are sort of the 'building blocks' that are used to build and renew cells, making them too important indeed.

Moreover, proteins are also involved in the production of blood, and helps with the creation of different hormones and antibodies.

As you must very well see by now, proteins are absolutely of the utmost importance, and for a childbearing woman, this importance must never be understated. If you aren't getting enough protein, your body may have trouble supplying your baby with the protein indispensable for its growth.

Essentially, you don't need to be stuffing yourself full of protein though – that would be excessive. Pregnant women only need 10 grams more protein than normal, or, 60 grams altogether (since the normal protein intake is about 50 grams).

And this can be acquired through a number of sources.

Some of the most common origin of protein include lean meats, poultry, fish, and dairy products. Although there are other sources too, the ones that we just mentioned are also the source of different other nutrients, which makes them all the more desirable.

Depending on your diet, you may even find that you don't need to willfully consume more protein. On average, Americans tend to consume more protein than they need anyway, and so you might already be getting enough, even with your pregnancy.

If you are vegetarian, your primary source of protein would be milk and eggs. But, for full fledged vegans, your only source of protein would be soy products.

Especially, this is not an issue, but vegans and vegetarians may have problems getting some of the other nutrients that they require when pregnant. Sometimes, it could be good to talk to a doctor or a nutritionist – but this guide should give you a great idea of what you are after!

All in all, you should have few issues getting the required dosage of protein.

Just as a further 'bonus', if you want a nice, sweet source of protein, why not try peanut butter!

Carbohydrates

Being your main source of energy, and so, also your baby's main source of energy, carbohydrates cannot be ignored or set aside.

True, may people opt for low-carb diets, but pregnancy is hardly the right time to cut back on your energy levels. Face it, you are going to need all the energy that you can get, so don't starve your body!

Furthermore, carbs also have important roles within various other bodily functions such as blood clotting, the immune system, and cell communication.

Fortunately, carbs are truly plentiful. Among the 'best' sources of carbs are: whole grains, fruits, vegetables, and dairy products. As you ought know by now, these are the 'best' sources because of the other nutrients that also come along with them, as part and parcel of the same food.

Depending on how active you are, your metabolism rate, and other factors, you will find that the 'ideal' carbohydrate intake varies. Almost, the recommended intake is 55% of the energy requirements of your body, which averages out to about 130 grams of carbs per day.

For pregnant women, the amount of carbohydrates that you should be rising in your daily diet is about 45 grams, making it a total of 175 grams.

A good rule to follow is to assign breakfast as the meal when you consume the most carbs. That way, you give your body energy after you wake up, and also ensure that you have ample time to work your way through the energy, so that there is little or no excess.

Later on, you will see that there exist a particular kind of carbs, i.e. folic acid enriched carbohydrates, which are going to be very beneficial too!

Fats

Although most people tend to shun away from the very word, fats are a very necessary part of nutrition.

For the most part, fats are a large energy source; that is evident from the high number of calories that they carry. But, when it comes to pregnant women, there is another consideration that should be made.

Some food types that contain fat also contain what are known as 'important fatty acids'. These are fatty acids that are not produced by the body, and hence, ought to be obtained in dietary form via food consumption.

And, as you may have guessed, some of these fundamental fatty acids are crucial for a baby's development, and are used in a variety of functions that range from transporting vitamins, right on to developing the nervous system of a baby.

So in short, you can't just cut out all fats from your diet completely!

Still, that being said, there are many types of fats, and it would be best if you try to stay away from saturated fats, and instead only go for the unsaturated variety. These 'unsaturated fats' can be found from a number of sources, including fish, nuts, and flaxseeds.

Some vegetable oils also carry unsaturated fats, though you should be careful to ensure that they don't contain those pesky 'trans fats' that are really something you would want to avoid due to the numerous problems they pose.

Try as hard as you can to keep your fat consumption anything from 20% to 30% of your total calorie intake.

One specific type of fat in particular, known as DHA, which is an omega-3 fatty acid, has been shown to actually play a great role in the development of a baby's brain and eyes. Commonly, it's found in oily fish, however nowadays you should have no problems locating supplements for it if you desire.

Note: The recommended intake for DHA is 200 milligrams daily.

All in all, by eating the right amount of saturated fats, you should be able to ensure that your baby is getting all the essential fatty acids that he or she requires!

Aside from these common nutrients that we've been discussing though, there are others, that really are going to be very necessary in order to ensure that your child has everything that he or she needs to develop, so let's move on to a class of nutrients that you should definitely know about…

Minerals

Granted, there are a lot of minerals out there, but when it comes to pregnancies, some are more important than others.

Different minerals tend to have vastly different functions, and it should come as no surprise that the minerals we're most interest in are those that tie in with development in some way or other.

These minerals, which are somehow connected with development, would naturally be needed in higher quantities than the norm during a pregnancy, as your baby will require them in order to grow in his or her own right!

To kick things off, let's start off with one of the most commonly known minerals that is tied to development…

1.   Calcium

Chances are, you already know that calcium is required to grow bones and teeth. Thus, babies require it too for exactly the same purpose!

Furthermore, calcium also plays a role in helping with the production of fluids for the lymphatic system. Don't worry if you don't know what that is – but just rest assured that calcium is of crucial importance.

Normally, the most readily available sources of calcium are dairy products, such as milk, yogurt, and cheese. Opt for the low-fat or no-fat varieties of these products if you like, so that you don't end up consuming too much fat.

Alternatively, you could skip the dairy products entirely, and go for very dark green leafy vegetables.

Nowadays, there are even a variety of calcium-enhanced juices, cereals, and so on, so you should have no trouble finding a good source of calcium that you can consume on a daily basis.

Overall, you should be getting about 1,000 mg of calcium a day for the duration of your pregnancy.

Bear in mind that, in tandem with calcium, you're going to need Vitamin D, which is irreplaceably important for the absorption of calcium. Later on we'll discuss this a little more, but essentially, Vitamin D is produced by the body in the presence of sunlight!

Anyway, now that we've discussed calcium, it's time we move on to another mineral…

2.   Iron

Yet another mineral that you probably recognize, iron is definitely a mineral that has such a large variety of tasks that it would be impossible to function without it.

Primarily, the most well known function of iron is its role in helping to carry oxygen through the blood, and delivering it to the entire body. Yes, that's just one example of how important iron is!

Other examples include the roles iron plays in the immunity system, metabolism, body temperature regulation, brain development, and so on.

For babies in particular, iron is irreplaceable as it is needed to help develop the circulatory system of your child.

Now, pregnant women already have an increased amount of blood flowing through their bodies compared to non-pregnant women. That means that already they need an increased amount of iron.

Fortunately, a lot of iron is conserved and reused, so the recommended quantity of iron intake for a pregnant woman is about 27 mg.

Getting that kind of iron content can be tough, depending on your diet. Some of the best sources of iron are various forms of meat, with red meat being an especially good source.

Poultry, fish, dark green leafy vegetables, eggs, and so on are also other sources, but it is worth noting that iron is not absorbed as well from eggs and vegetarian food as it is from meat.

Therefore, if you're a vegetarian you'll find that you need to consume a larger quantity of such foods to get the required iron content. Eating foods high in Vitamin C can help increase the amount of iron you absorb, but even then, it doesn't compare to that of meat.

If you find that you're unable to get enough iron in your system, for whatever reason, you should definitely start taking supplements. Honestly, your baby needs the iron, as do you, or you risk developing a whole lot of problems, including anemia.

What we've covered so far are the most important minerals out there for pregnant women. Do be aware though that, as a part of a balanced diet, you should really be consuming more than just these minerals.

Still, during a pregnancy, these are definitely the ones that you want to be absolutely certain that you're taking enough of. Time to move on to our next nutrient…

Folic Acid

Remember us mentioning this earlier when we talked about carbohydrates? Well, even if you don't, no need to fret.

Folic acid, or folate, as it is sometimes called, is really just a type of Vitamin B. Normally, the body requires it to help replicate DNA as well as produce and maintain new cells. As you can probably notice, these are things that would be very important during any pregnancy!

By ensuring that you're getting enough folic acid, you could avoid a number of very serious problems, most of which involve neural tube defects such as spina bifida, or even birth defects involving the brain and spinal cord.

Unfortunately, many pregnant women do not actually end up getting enough folic acid from natural sources (about 40 milligrams is the standard requirement).

Sources of folic acid include things such as dark, green and leafy vegetables, dark and brightly colored fruits, beans, peas, and even nuts. However, even if you do eat some of these kinds of foods, chances are you aren't eating enough of them to fulfill your folic acid needs.

One way to overcome this lack of folic acid is to simply consume a multivitamin, most of which will give you the required 40 milligrams of folic acid. That way you can rest easy, knowing that you're on top of things.

Start to be sure that you're getting enough folic acid before your pregnancy, so that from the very first moment of conception, your baby's risks are lessened!

Other Vitamins

In tandem with the specific case of folic acid, there are other vitamins that are also going to play roles in the development of your baby.

Since vitamins are such a diverse bunch, the roles they play are equally diverse, so let's look at them one by one - or at least, hit the big ones that you should be aware of:

1.   Vitamin A

On the whole Vitamin A has a number of uses within the body, including such things that involve healthy skin, bone growth, as well as eyesight. All these things are going to help with your baby's development.

Carrots are the best sources for Vitamin A, but apart from that, you could find it in ample quantities within dark leafy green vegetables, and even sweet potatoes.

2.   Vitamin C

Earlier we had touched on how Vitamin C can help iron absorption from vegetables. Really, it also has other uses, including helping with the health of the gums, teeth, and bones, and also has its own role to play in fighting infections

Normally, the single best source of Vitamin C would be citrus-y fruit, and you definitely want to be sure you are taking enough of it (about 80 milligrams daily).

3.   Vitamin B6

Vitamin B6 has the important task of helping with metabolize proteins, fats and carbohydrates, and also help form red blood cells too.

But, during pregnancy, the role that Vitamin B6 plays is absolutely enhanced, as it has been found to be required to help develop the brain and nervous system within unborn children.

Some of the best sources for Vitamin B6 include pork, ham, whole-grains, and bananas.

4.   Vitamin D

Once again, we had touched on this earlier when we mentioned how Vitamin D was needed to absorb calcium. That aside, it also, helps with the formation of teeth and bones, which is too much necessary for a child's growth.

Fortunately, as you previously know, the body produces Vitamin D of its own accord, when exposed to sunlight.

So all you need to do is ensure that you are not cloistering yourself indoors and that you are really getting a little sunlight here and there; and you ought to be fine!

By now you should have a good idea of what you need to do in order to obtain sufficient vitamins for a nutritious diet.

All in all, none of what we have covered so far is really anything too out of the ordinary, and must not require you to even modify your diet that much (unless, your existing diet was completely unhealthy).

Speaking of unhealthy diets, even though you now know most of the fundamentals of nutrition during pregnancy, there is still something else to consider: All the bad things that you should avoid such as the plague.

Let's take a look at those right now!

Food and Substances worth Avoiding During Pregnancy

As part and parcel of getting all the right food during pregnancy, you will also want to avoid the wrong kinds of foods and substances.

What are the wrong types of foods and substances? Well, there are a lot of things out there that have been proven to adversely impact pregnancy, and sadly, some of these things are commonly found in the diets of many people.

And even more unfortunately, some of substances are actually quite addictive, as you will soon see. That makes them even harder to avoid, but there are several compelling reasons why you should still try.

Anyway, without further delay, let's start looking at the specific types of food and substances that we're talking about.

Alcohol

Odds are, you probably did expect alcohol to feature in this list, and really it does occupy the very top spot.

Naturally, the more general ill-effects of alcohol are well documented, but when it comes to pregnancy, there are some very specific side effects that come with drinking alcohol and they are definitely the kind of thing that you'd want to avoid.

For one, alcohol has been substantially linked with causing birth defects, which can range from very mild, but in some cases could even be severe.

Really, the list of such defects is pretty long, and includes things from mental retardation, right on to defects involving the heart, face, and other parts of the body. In short you do not want to risk such things happening.

At the current point in time, there is no real data as to how much alcohol is 'safe' for consumption, which is why the good way to go about things is to just avoid all alcohol for the duration of your pregnancy.

If you have been consuming small amounts of alcohol before you found out you were pregnant, don't worry too much. Just be sure to stop as soon as possible.

Bottom line, it's worth becoming a teetotaler for your child's sake during your pregnancy!

Caffeine

Next up as far as things to avoid are concerned is caffeine, which, as you probably know is widely found in a number of drinks. Yes, that's right, it is not just coffee that contains caffeine; even things like tea, soft drinks, and some chocolates can have more than their fair share of caffeine.

Unlike alcohol though, you don't need to lay off caffeine completely, unless you truly want to, that is.

Basically, caffeine is completely safe, as long as you are consuming it in moderate amounts. Incidentally, the standard definition for moderate caffeine consumption is about 300 milligrams in a day, which amounts to about 3 cups of coffee, or thereabouts.

Going above this limit, but can cause unwanted side effects, including birth defects.

Assuming you regularly consume a large amount of caffeine on a daily basis, it can be hard to kick the habit, so you will want to start quickly and cut down until you are within the 'safe zone'.

Even after your baby is born, if you are breastfeeding, you will still want to keep your caffeine intake to a minimum. Largely, this is due to caffeine that could transfer to your baby through your breast milk, and lead to countless other issues.

All things said and done, as long as you are able to cut back, by hook or by crook, you should have very few problems with caffeine. Try reducing coffee slowly, initially, if you have issues reducing the actual amount that you drink.

Mainly, these 2 substances (caffeine and alcohol), are the primary types of food that you should avoid. Apart from these though, there are other things that you might want to be careful about, but for a very different reason, as you are about to see…

Food Safety during Pregnancy

Knowing the right food to eat is a good start, but you must still be careful. Nutrition, and the adverse affects of some foods are both cornerstones of good eating for a pregnancy, however there is one more risk that needs to be addressed.

This risk takes the form of food-borne diseases.

While at normal times, you may not be very concerned about food-borne diseases, unless they are very risky, during a pregnancy it is not just you that you have to worry about – you will also undoubtedly be worried about your unborn child.

And unlike you, your child when exposed to certain diseases, could end up suffering side effects that you may not even realize exist.

When it comes to food safety, there really is no such thing as being too safe, and knowing what to look out for, avoid, and how to go about food safety in general, is going to be a tremendous asset on your part.

Here are some of the risky diseases that you should be aware of:

Listeriosis

As a disease, it is spread by a form of bacteria, and is found in earth and groundwater, and therefore also commonly located on plants. More concerning however is the fact that this bacteria is also very often found in many refrigerated products.

At first, if you have listeriosis, you may not even notice it. Mostly, it would pass itself off as a type of common flu, and you'll end up having a fever, chills, and maybe even diarrhea.

However, as the disease progresses, it could even affect the nervous system, and cause headaches, stiff neck, confusion, balance issues, and so on.

While this is all very unpleasant, the risk that manifests itself during pregnancy is worse.

Listeriosis very often results in miscarriage or premature birth. In some cases, it can even lead to fetal death or cause a severe illness in the newborn that could be fatal too.

Basically even if the baby is born, safely, it doesn't mean that the risk goes away. When a baby is prematurely born especially, he or she is bound to be much more susceptible to the continuing illness, and the risk is very real indeed.

Toxoplasmosis

As yet another very real risk, toxoplasmosis is a parasite that is spread through food.

Overall, its risk is most apparent in the fact that it can cause many health problems in unborn children, the more serious of which include mental retardation, and even blindness. For most grown-ups however, they may even have been infected before, and simply not noticed it or built up an immunity too it.

Bear in mind though, that this immunity may not extend to your child, and so you need to treat this disease seriously.

Mercury Poisoning

Last, but certainly not least, there is the question of mercury poisoning. Most people don't even really think this is a legitimate risk since, after all – we're not really exposed to mercury all that often, are we?

Well, the truth is – we are.

Some types of fish contain some pretty high levels of mercury, and so if you're eating these kinds of fish, you can get quite a bit of mercury in your body. While it may not be enough to harm you, it could harm your child.

Notably, mercury is known to cause defects in a developing nervous system.

Frankly speaking though, this is one of the easier risks to avoid seeing as the types of fish that normally can have dangerous levels of mercury are rarely staple foods in any diet. These fish include: king mackerel, tilefish, shark, and swordfish.

So, if you happen to have a taste for any of those, you may want to consider laying off them for the time being, at least until your child is born.

Food Safety Measures

Great, so mercury poisoning can be avoided by dodging certain types of fish, but what about the other two diseases that we discussed?

Frankly speaking, they're not too hard to avoid too, and all you need is to be aware of a few simple, basic, and really straightforward food safety measures that you can implement. By doing so, you'll reduce your risk of contracting such diseases to being practically nonexistent!

Here's a list of what you should do:

1.	Cook food thoroughly at the recommended temperature.

2.	Peel or thoroughly wash any and all fruits and vegetables during preparation.

3.	Avoid all food that contains unpasteurized milk

4.	Avoid refrigerated foods that are 'uncooked' or 'partially uncooked' such as pate, spreads, and smoked seafood.

5.   Do not eat frozen hot dogs, luncheon meat, or deli meat unless they're cooked properly and fully.

Simple enough isn't it? All of these steps combined should dramatically reduce your chances of ever having to face either listeriosis or toxoplasmosis. And at the same time, this means that your babies are going to be subjected to a lot less risk too!

Effectively, this completes your journey through discovering what you should, or should not, be eating during a pregnancy. In just a few words, we'll leave you to go ahead and start applying everything that we've covered.

Final Words on Eating Right during Pregnancy

Although our approach has been centered on the idea of eating with pregnancy in mind, you will find that a lot of what we have discussed is really beneficial to you at other times too.

Still, just to recap, let's go over some of the major points of this guide:

1.   First, you found out that 'eating for two' does not exactly mean eating for two, and know about calories and weight gain during pregnancy

2.   Next, we went over nutrition, comprehensively cataloging what you must or must not be eating

3.   After that, you delved into some substances that must be avoided at all costs, or at least reduced

4.   Finally, we discussed food safety to protect you from food borne diseases while you're pregnant

All that sound about right? If some of it does not seem to ring a bell, then go ahead and refer back to the previous pages!

End of the day, with the right food and nutrition during pregnancy, your baby will be healthier, and happier!

Good luck with it all!

CHAPTER THREE

Absolutely Everything You Need to Know About Labor and Delivery

Are you ready to give birth?

If you are pregnant, it is highly likely that you have asked yourself very question before. Sure, getting pregnant may have been tough, however from what you have heard, you undoubtedly know that going through labor can be tougher still in a different way.

Admittedly, it is a satisfying and beautiful experience. That much should go without saying.

However still, it is a trying experience too, and one that you must definitely be as prepared for as possible.

Bearing this in mind, let's ask that same question again: Are you ready to give birth? Do you know what you should know about delivery? Do you know what you must do when you go into labor?

Many people are inclined to think that everything will just fall into place when the time comes. While that can happen, the truth is that it helps to be fully prepared so that you can be completely certain that everything is going to fall into place, and not have to face the prospect of anything going wrong.

Being confident, well informed, and fully supported, you will find that child labor can truly be one of the most memorable and rewarding experiences of your lifetime.

That's what this guide is going to aim to provide for you – all the information that you need to overcome every uncertainty that you may have about labor and delivery. So when the time finally does come, you will know how to recognize it, and exactly what to do!

Of course, this doesn't mean that you must forego any childbirth education classes that you may be taking. They too can help you, and provide you with some practical exercises that would be beneficial in the long run.

Still, now that you have this guide in your hand, you are off to a flying start.

Chances are, you fully expected that the very first thing we'd discuss is labor itself, and that discussion is going to take us to a period in time that is actually right before you actually go into labor.

Why are we looking at what happens before you go into labor? Well, you are about to find out in this next section!

Identifying the Signs and Symptoms of Pre-Labor

Deep into your third trimester, your body is already preparing itself for the labor that it knows is about to pursue.

Due to this, there are many changes, both noticeable and unnoticeable, that will occur. And, as a direct result of these changes, you might even sometimes mistake some of them to be the signs that you are going into labor.

False alarms such as this, while common, are something that you will want to avoid.

Each and every time that you feel you are going into labor, it automatically gives you a sense of urgency and you will want to get everything sorted and rush off to the hospital. When this happens due to a false alarm, it can be quite tedious.

Imagine if you had numerous false alarms, as you very well may end up having!

Honestly, it isn't too difficult to spot the differences between the false alarms, and real labor, if you know what to look out for. That's why we are kicking this guide off during the timeline right before actual labor occurs.

By doing so, you should be able to grasp exactly what your body is going through, and be able to pinpoint the difference between what are just natural bodily changes, and actual labor.

Understanding this difference is the main drive of this section. Shall we get started?

Symptoms in the Days and Weeks Leading Up to Labor

Within the third trimester, you will eventually find yourself facing various symptoms and signs that will help you to know that your due date is fast approaching.

Admittedly, these signs vary from person to person, but if you are able to know and understand them, then you must be able to spot at least one or two, which will then give you an inkling of just how soon you may go into labor.

Most notable among these symptoms is the one known as 'lightening' or 'dropping'.

In short, lightening occurs when your tummy seems to descend into the pelvis, lightening the load on your upper abdomen. For some mothers, this is a very obvious change, but in others it could be almost unnoticeable.

As a result of this lightening however, you can expect that you will sense yourself carrying your baby differently, and also may find that the urge to pass urine comes stronger and more frequently, due to the increased pressure at the pelvic area.

Also, this increased pressure can cause cramps, groin pain, and even a constant lower backache.

Coupled with this, all the other changes in your body can cause several other symptoms.

For one thing, you can expect to lose some weight during this period, the amount of water your body retains is going to fluctuate. In some cases, you may find that you don't actually lose weight, but gain weight more slowly than previously.

Furthermore, you are going to have a lot of hormonal changes, and can expect your energy levels to soar and dip at the drop of a penny. Sometimes, these soaring and dipping energy levels may be accompanied by various urges, to do things like prepare for your baby's arrival.

Finally, there are the more solid evidences of next labor, and these include:

1.   Passage of the mucus plug

During your pregnancy, there has been a thick wad of mucus that has sealed off your cervix, to protect your baby from infections that may travel through it.

Chances are, you didn't even know it was there, but as your delivery date approaches, you can expect that it will become dislodged, when your cervix begins to dilate. Mind you, this can occur anything from a few days before labor, to the point right at labor itself.

Many people feel that this is a firm indication that you are about to go into labor, but this really isn't the case. So even if you do notice the passage of the mucus plug, don't panic, you may not be in labor for quite some time still.

2.   Pink show

During the dilation of the cervix that we just mentioned, some unfortunate side effects can be experienced, and the most common among these is the rupturing of some of the blood capillaries that lace the surface of the cervix itself.

While this isn't a big problem, it can manifest itself physically by a small amount of 'pink show', or bleeding.

Once again, the dilation of the cervix can occur anywhere from right before, up to a few days before, labor, so it doesn't mean that you are in labor, just that you will be soon enough.

Both of these two signs indicate the labor is going to happen soon. However, it is still a very subjective measure, and varies from person to person, so you are not going to be able to gauge exactly how soon it will be before you are actually in labor.

Furthermore, there is one other symptom that you will face that serves to more than confuse the situation…

Braxton Hick Contractions

Mainly, this is the cause of the so-called 'false labor' self-diagnosis that many pregnant women face.

Essentially, Braxton Hick contractions are meant to be 'practice' contractions, or rather, the body's way of getting ready for the actual event itself. Unfortunately, unless you have been through labor before, it is understandable that you could find it hard to differentiate between these practice contractions, and the real thing.

Although some people say that there are readily apparent differences, the truth is that despite being billed as 'practice' contractions, Braxton Hick contractions can appear to be just as intense, and just as painful.

Add to that the fact that you have no benchmark to compare it against, and it must be easy to see why things can become rather confused.

Certainly, you don't wish to be precipitate to the hospital, or getting started for what amounts to a false labor. Keeping this in mind, it is crucial that you learn the difference between Braxton Hick contractions and the real thing.

Some ways to pinpoint if or not your contractions are a sign of labor, or simply Braxton Hick contractions include:

1.   Regularity and frequency of contractions

'Real' labor implies of contractions that rise in frequency, regularity, and intensity.

In other words, this means that you are going to be able to spot a pattern emerging, where the time between your contractions is steadily reducing, and they're getting longer, stronger, and more painful.

If this isn't the case, then chances are, your contractions are of the Braxton Hick variety.

2.   Subsiding contractions

Should your contractions ultimately subside, which means that they were evidently Braxton Hick contractions?

To check this out, try changing your position, or even drinking two glasses of water or some other (non-alcoholic!) beverage. Admittedly, this doesn't always work, but it is a good thing to try, just to be sure.

3.   Center of pain

For some women, Braxton Hick contractions are accompanied by pain that is noticeably centered in the lower abdomen, as opposed to the lower back (where 'real' contractions would be).

Through these signs you must be able to safely identify the difference. Still, don't feel bad if you are unable to, for some women, false labor really can convincingly appear to be real labor, and so it may be close to impossible to differentiate.

Similarly, it is worth keeping in mind that for some women, their real labor could seem to be a false labor, and that's why you have undoubtedly heard the stories of women being surprised when their baby just 'pops out' while they're out shopping!

With what you know now though, you are as prepared as possible to identify pre-labor when it occurs.

So now, let's move on to the real thing!

Starting to go into Labor: What you should do? And How to handle it!

When you do go into labor for real, it can be a pretty daunting affair. Almost immediately, you will recognize that you have to get so many things sorted out, and trying to do everything at once can cause you to panic.

Remember: Don't panic! Try to keep as calm and composed as possible so that you are able to do everything that you need to do.

To this end, there are several steps that you can take to ensure that everything is prepared for when you go into labor. Let's take a minute to go over some of these things…

Preparation for Labor

Right from the moment that you are pregnant, you know that eventually, you will end up delivering your child. So, essentially, you must have a whole 9 months to prepare everything and get ready for when it actually happens.

Even if you are already well along in your pregnancy, it is never too late, and you will find that most of the preparation that you need for your labor and delivery is really pretty basic.

Right now, we are going to give you an insight into the exact preparation that you will need:

1.   Be sure to arrange your caregiver. Essentially, your caregiver could be your husband, or could even be your mother, or anyone else close to you who is going to help you through your labor.

2.   Plan ahead as to whether you are going to be delivering at home, with the help of a midwife, or going to the hospital.

3.   If you are delivering with the help of a midwife, be sure to have their number somewhere that is easily accessible.

4.   If you are delivering at a hospital, be sure that both you and your caregiver know the best way to get there, alternative routes if necessary (to avoid rush hour traffic and so on), as well as where the best car park is. Also, be certain that your doctor's phone number is somewhere accessible, and that you have done all the required paperwork well in advance too.

5.   Assuming you have other children, you must prearrange for someone willing to come in and take care of them at a moments notice.

Now, you should notice that none of these steps are anything too complicated, and indeed, you must be able to do them without too much hassle.

Ideally, your caregiver must be the person that you trust and want by your side throughout the entire process. He or she is going to be a form of support for you, so you should definitely choose wisely.

Also, your caregiver must know what labor consists of, and be able to help you along as much as possible!

Preparing this well in advance is going to help ensure that your entire delivery goes as smoothly as possible. But we are getting slightly ahead of ourselves at this stage…

Although you may know how to identify real labor already, it is important that we establish just when exactly you should be calling your caregiver and midwife or doctor. Admittedly, if you really are in labor there's no such thing as 'too early', but it would still help to have some idea of what to expect…

What to Do When Labor Starts…

Based on what we discussed earlier about Braxton Hick contractions, you must already have a good idea of what 'real' contractions are going to be like. In a nutshell though, they're going to be increasing in intensity, frequency, and length.

Still, there are no hard and fast rules as to exactly when you should begin to call your caregiver. Needless to say, it will be a while before you are able to determine that it really is time for your baby to be delivered, so it would be helpful to have a rough guideline.

These are some things that you must consider, but do remember that it really is very subjective:

1.   5-Minute apart contractions

As a rule of thumb, it is time to start getting things in motion when you start to have contractions that are 5 minutes apart. Timing your contractions is, of course, part and parcel of determining that you are really in labor, so once you reach this point, it is time to get going.

Mind you, it wouldn't hurt to do it sooner, even at the point when the contractions are 10 minutes apart. This is due to the fact that some women do have very rapid labors, and their contractions can increase in frequency very quickly.

Similarly, if you have a long trip to your hospital, or your midwife will take time to get there, you might want to start earlier than usual.

2.   When your water breaks

If your water has broken already, that means that you really are quite close to delivery, and you should immediately start to your preplanned arrangements.

In some situations, the fluid may be stained a dark, greenish-brown color, and if so, you must act quickly because your baby could be in distress. Remember not to panic though, the best thing to do is to take action calmly!

3.   Vaginal bleeding

You must look at vaginal bleeding (not just a pink show), it could be an indication of a premature separation of the placenta. Once again, don't worry, this is a simple problem that doctors can deal with, but it's imperative that you get to the hospital as fast as possible.

Anyway, once you have identified these signs, and know that you must be getting things in motion – all that remains is to put your plans into action. Call up those people that you must call up, primarily your caregiver, doctor or midwife, and anyone else who is going to help you take care of things.

Then, go to the hospital, or wait for your midwife to arrive. Now that you are in labor, this is where the real trying part begins…

Facing Both Labor and Delivery

Despite the fact that, now, you must be at the hospital and have professional care, or with your midwife, who essentially amounts to the same thing – you are really just getting to the tough part!

Honestly speaking, labor can last quite a long time.

For first time mothers, the average amount of time spent in labor is anything from 12 to 18 hours! Yes, that is pretty much half a day or more!

Admittedly, you won't be at hospital for most of this time, seeing as you would have been timing your contractions and only headed over when they were 5 to 10 minutes apart. Still, even by doing that, you could still be waiting for hours in the hospital before you actually deliver.

So that you know exactly what you are go to be facing, let's go over the four main stages of labor and deliver.

First Stage

This first stage starts when your contractions do. From that point onwards, you are officially in labor, but as you know, the vast majority of this time will be spent away from the hospital, until your contractions are 5 to 10 minutes apart.

Originally, the brunt of labor will not hit you. When the contractions are rather mild, and spaced out, you will have plenty of time to rest and relax in between, especially when the spacing between contractions is more than 20 minutes.

So simply go about your normal schedule, and occupy yourself till the window closes. When it does, head over to the hospital, call your midwife.

Progressively, as your contractions coming the five-minutes-apart threshold, things will be getting more serious. At this stage, you will undoubtedly be realizing that your baby is about to come out, soon, and you will be mentally preparing yourself for the trials ahead!

Still, 5 minutes in between contractions does give you some time to wait, so use that time to do what you need to do – go to the bathroom, have a drink, and try to relax, maybe read a magazine or talk to your partner.

Some women, at this moment, start taking different forms of pain relief, which your doctor or midwife must be able to afford. Others choose to not take any kind of pain relief, and the choice is definitely up to you.

Finally, at the tail end of stage one, you are going to face one of the hardest portions of your labor. By now, the contractions you are facing will be about 2 to 3 minutes apart, and last up to a minute and a half or more. That means that you are going to just have mere seconds in between contractions.

Sometimes this stage can last up to an hour or more, so be prepared!

At this time, it's very normal if you feel nauseous and vomit. Don't be afraid about it, and it is just part of your body's reflex to being in labor.

Whoever your caregiver is, they must be aware of this trying time during your labor, and this is when any and all support they can offer is most crucial. You will need all the backing and encouragement that you can get!

Try to get into as comfortable a position as possible, and in the few seconds of break you have in between contractions, sip cold water. Hang in there, no matter what!

Be aware that this stage officially ends the minute you become fully dilated, and that means that from there on out, you are officially delivering your baby!

Second Stage

Many individuals refer to this stage as the 'pushing' stage, because it begins when you are wholly dilated, and ready to give birth, and ends when your baby has been fully delivered!

In general, this second stage could perhaps last for up to four hours. Yes, that is a prolonged time, but it rarely tends to run that long for most women, while it does differ on a case to case basis.

Also, belong on the medications that you are taking, your position, and your baby's position, the length of time it takes could be either shorter or longer.

Of course, such things as C-sections do not fall under this umbrella at all.

Anyway, assuming you are going about it the 'old fashioned' way, and pushing, there are several things that you can do to smooth things along and help yourself and your child!

1.   No contractions after dilation

Sometimes, after you are dilated, your contractions suddenly subside and go away for a period of time. Don't worry if they do, this is a absolutely natural occurrence.

Occasionally, this 'rest and relax' phase as it is termed, could take for as long as 1 hour.

Theoretically, this lapse in contractions exists so that the mother can gather her strength, and the baby can get into position. Some hospitals recommend that you try to push harder even during this period, but that is not actually necessary.

Best advice: Just sit back, relax, and wait for the contractions to come back.

2.   Getting into position

Now that your baby is ready to come out into the world, you should be getting into the best position possible to help him or her do just that!

Modern birth beds can be adjusted to accommodate a wide range of positions, and the best ones are those where you are at least relatively 'upright' so that gravity helps the process along.

Some mothers find this too uncomfortable though, in which case the more traditional 'lying-down' positions are fine.

Normally, you would have talked to your doctor, midwife, or anyone else who is assisting you, and determined the position that you'd like to give birth in well in advance of this point in time.

End of the day, it is up to you!

3.   Pushing urges

Some mothers end up feeling an almost out of control urge to push. Others don't feel anything.

Depending on your circumstances, you may find that it is impossible to fight versus the urge to push, and by this stage you mustn't. Actually, this is the more 'natural' type of childbirth, where your body tells you when to push, and you do so.

However, for women who don't feel the urge to push at all, there are other options.

This includes 'hold your breath' technique, or 'purple pushing', as it is otherwise known. Basically, purple pushing consists of holding your breathing to the count of ten over contractions, while pushing.

Whereas, as you would wait for, your doctor or midwife will give you some advices as to when and how to push, it is definitely something that you ought to discuss beforehand.

When purple pushing do not hold your breath for more than a 10-count. What you are trying to accomplish is to help along the 'push', but you don't want to starve your body, and baby, of oxygen in the process!

4.   No time limits on pushing

Although classic birth coaching does advise that you push whenever possible, the truth is that it really isn't necessary. We now know for a fact that forcing pushes doesn't really help you deliver that much faster – the difference is a few minutes, at very most.

So therefore, you can request of your doctor or midwife that there be no time limits placed on your pushing, so long as both you and your baby are doing well.

That way, although delivery might take just a little longer, you are also cutting down the risk of meconium stained amniotic fluid – which can cause your baby to go into distress.

Everything said and done, as long as anesthesia isn't used, and as long as your baby is fine, there is no real reason to impose a time limit on yourself. Sure, you might want to not make this stage last too long, but that should be entirely up to you, and you can decide to push at your own comfort level.

Knowing all of this about pushing, you should be able to get through this second stage with little or no problem. Of course, your caregiver should be there, supporting you every step of the way, and you are going to be grateful for that help.

Normally, the baby is born headfirst, and as his head begins to crest, and finally the rest of the body emerges, that is the end of this second stage of labor.

Naturally, you are probably wondering, "So, what's left after this?", and many individuals do, but the reality is that there is at least one more formal stage to childbirth, more informal stage too!

Third Stage

When compared against the two other stages that we have already discussed, this third stage really is a 'mini' stage.

As we said before, by now, your baby has already been delivered, and opportunities are you may actually even be holding him in your arms for the first time, which is a joyous moment for every mother!

So when you are asked to push again, the first thing to cross your mind would undoubtedly be, "Why?"

And the answer to that is easy: Even though your baby has been delivered, you need to expel again another thing from your body: The placenta.

Admittedly, pushing the placenta out is too much easier than the process of delivering your baby. In some cases, it could take up to one hour, while for most women, it takes just a minutes.

Seeing as the 'push' involved this time is too much easier, you don't need to concern yourself a lot with it, and can actually just afford to concentrate on your baby. Do not let the fact that your work isn't over spoil this very wonderful moment of bonding!

Some evidence suggests that nursing your baby will help the uterus contract naturally and expel the placenta. If you plan to breastfeed, even if just initially, this certainly isn't going to hurt, and so you might as well try it.

With your baby in your arms now, the three official stages of labor are over. But, as we did mention, there is a fourth 'unofficial' stage…

Fourth (Unofficial) Stage

Mind you, the reason this stage of labor is considered unofficial is because, now that your baby has been delivered, and your placenta expelled, there really aren't going to be any more contractions.

But now, after childbirth, known differently as the 'postpartum' stage, is unofficially accepted as the fourth stage of labor, despite its lack of contractions.

Also, this stage isn'trt without its own tribulations.

All things said and done, now that your child has entered this world, and is in your arms, you are really entering a new stage of your life. Understandably, you are going to be feeling a mix of emotions, and although happiness and joy tend to be overwhelming at the start, gradually, they are going to give way to apprehension and uncertainty.

Don't feel guilty about this – it is only natural to worry, and as a parent, you are going to find that you are bound to worry a whole lot more than you did previously!

At the same time, your body is also undergoing changes of its own. Having changed in so many ways to accommodate your pregnancy, it is now facing a reversal, and going back to be close to the way that it once was.

During this time, a lot of things are happening at once, externally and internally, and so you can expect that you are going to be affected in more ways that one.

Among the trials of this period, nothing is more evident than that of postpartum depression.

Many things are linked in to cause it, and they range from such things as hormonal imbalances due to your condition, right down to conflicts, stress, and a difficulty with adjusting to changes.

Really – the list of possible factors is a long one, and encompasses most everything that you'd naturally go through after a pregnancy.

So many women go through postpartum depression of some form or other, though in most cases it is pretty mild. Sometimes though, some mothers find themselves faced with more severe cases of postpartum depression, and it's in situations like that where you must surely get help.

Do not take postpartum depression lightly. It can, quite clearly, develop into a disorder and cause a host of other issues.

Whereas feeling down occasionally is normal, and natural, if you find that it is spiraling out of control you ought to fast let others know, and seek medical help. Nip off the problem rapidly, so that it doesn't get to the point where you are unable to function due to being so severely depressed. Yes, in some cases postpartum depression can be so serious that leads to mental breakdowns.

Anyway, now that you are aware of the risk, you know that it is something to look out for. Be sure to let your partner know too, as he is going to be a support that you definitely require, and could help you when you feel down.

Apart from that, this fourth stage is really something that you will find yourself easing into, slowly but surely.

One thing that absolutely helps is to be ready for your child right from the start. That means that you must have sorted out before you go into labor, so that by the time you have delivered your baby, and are ready to go house, you can be confident that everything is sorted out and awaiting your arrival.

With that, your labor and delivery is done, and you are pretty much at the last legs of your journey. Granted – an even bigger journey awaits you, and that is the journey of motherhood that is going to last you the rest of your lifetime!

Getting ready for that, and learning about it, is another story though.

Final Words on Labor and Delivery

Do you feel like you now know everything you need to know about labor and delivery? Well, you should! Over the course of this guide, we have walked you through absolutely everything – starting right from the very beginning, in the days leading up to labor, and ending with the delivery of your child, and a few days after that!

In essence, you now ought to have a strong grasp of the total picture.

As you read this guide, you may have noticed several points of interest that stuck with you, but it really is necessary that you remember that each point made is really just part of the bigger whole.

Let's go over some of the highlights of what we have covered, just to be certain that you are on top of everything:

1.   First, we started off by looking into some of the signs and symptoms that start a few days before labor.

2.   Then, we looked at 'false labor' and how to distinguish Braxton Hick contractions from 'real' contractions.

3.   After that, we delved into labor itself, and what you must do to prepare for it, as well as how you must handle it when it begins.

4.   Then, we explored the three official stages of labor, making certain that you know what to expect in each and every one.

5.   We also covered some of the fundamental 'need to know' aspects of pushing during labor.

6.   Last, we dealt with the final 'unofficial' fourth stage of labor, and you must know the danger of postpartum depression now too.

If any of what we just mentioned sounds unfamiliar, then you should be leafing back through the pages before this one, and reading up on what you might have missed out on!

Equipped with the knowledge that you now have, you will find that you aren't likely to get thrown any 'curveballs' during your labor, and you should be able to face it wholly aware of everything that's going on, and how to prepare and deal with it fully.

Good luck!

CHAPTER FOUR

Everything You Need to Know About Getting Started with Prenatal Workouts

Pregnancy is a trying time. Apart from all the changes that your body is going through, from physical changes right down to hormonal changes, you are also going to be struggling to get used to the lifestyle changes that you are forced to adapt.

Keeping this in mind, it is no surprise that many people get so caught up in what they're going through, that they unknowingly change their lifestyles more than they should.

In no way is this more evident than in the area of exercise.

Naturally, this depends a lot on the type of person you are. Supposing you were the type that used to get a lot of exercise, then this is going to be a great change to your lifestyle, but it is still one that popularly happens.

But, if you were an individual that was already fairly sedentary, then the change to a slightly more sedentary lifestyle can frequently go unnoticed.

Either way, as you are about to find out, slipping into a sedentary lifestyle, without much exercise, isn't a good thing. While it may seem tempting – resisting that temptation is really one of the best things that you can do!

Soon, you will see why this is the case.

After that, this guide is going to give you everything you need to know to get started with your own prenatal workouts, so that you don't risk lapsing!

Without any delay, let's just jump straight into things, and introduce you to the ideas of prenatal workouts.

Introduction to Prenatal Workouts

By this point, it must go without saying that prenatal workouts are really just, as the name implies, any and all workouts that you carry out during a pregnancy, and before you give birth.

Sometimes, people even use the term to describe workouts that are carried out post- pregnancy, but this isn't the case at all. In fact, as you will see soon, there is a distinct difference between the type of workouts we are discussing and the ones that would be carried out after pregnancy.

Largely, this is due to the fact that post-pregnancy, you are going to be able to gradually go back to a more 'regular' workout schedule.

However during your pregnancy, you will instead find that you have various limitations as to what you can do. After all, you are carrying a child, and each and every workout that you undertake should take that into account.

So while you do want to be getting some exercise, you definitely don't want to push yourself too far, or do anything that might be bad for your unborn baby.

Of course, this begs a question, and that is, "Why would you want to be getting any exercise at all? Wouldn't it be safer to just wait until after you have delivered and then get back to a regular workout routine?"

Once again, this ties in with the importance of prenatal workouts, and it is a topic that we are going to discuss right now!

Important Role of Prenatal Workouts

Naturally, exercising keeps you fit. That much is something that you are probably intimately aware of, but you must understand that 'being fit' has a great importance to your pregnancy.

Once you commit to a prenatal workout program, your principal concern is not going to be to stay trim, or tone up muscles, or even rise your stamina. Of course, these will all be benefits that you obtain anyway but they aren't the focus that you are aiming for.

Instead, what you ought to be most affected with, are those related to your pregnancy itself!

In this, prenatal workouts come to the fore because, if carried out correctly, they can rise your level of comfort over your pregnancy, and can even ease your experience over delivery.

Even after pregnancy, the benefits of exercising continue to manifest themselves, most notably by reducing your risk of undergoing postpartum depression.

Anyway, to give you a good idea of why you must definitely be starting to think about a prenatal workout program, here are some of the important benefits that you can expect to obtain if you do:

1.   Good flexibility and great blood circulation that will rise your comfort over pregnancy and ensure that you do not suffer from many muscle pains.

2.   Less water retention, stress, weight gains and tension will further reduce discomfort that many pregnant women face.

3.   Stretch marks and varicose veins will loom up slowly.

4.   The risk of abdominal separation, where the abdominal muscles 'part' from each other due to the increase in the size of the belly, will be far less.

5.   Calcium absorption will happen at good rate, helping ensure that both you and your baby are getting quantities that are required.

6.   Stamina, fitness, and overall strength and muscle control will be enhanced.

See how important prenatal workouts are? Simply by spending a few time on a regular routine, you could end up finding that many common issues women face over pregnancy are alleviated.

Overall, this will ease your way through your pregnancy, and help you to face it without suffering much at all!

And bear in mind, what we have discussed are, for the most part, just the physical advantages of prenatal workout programs.

By exercising regularly, you are going to be also promoting a feeling of well being, boosting your confidence, and helping yourself build a more positive self image. Let's face it, we all need this, especially during pregnancy when it is so easy to become depressed at the changes that our bodies are going through.

Now that you know just how a regular workout program can help you, how about we start getting into the meat of this guide.

No – we are not going to go through the exact exercises that you could be carrying out just yet, because before we begin that it is important that you know where you must start, and what you should prepare beforehand…

Complete Preparation for Prenatal Workouts

Okay so before we begin this, let's establish one thing: you are pregnant yes, but that doesn't mean you are fragile. At the same time though, it does mean that your body is undergoing a lot of changes, and you are carrying another life within you – so you can't exactly be reckless about what you do either!

That's the key to prenatal exercise preparation really: Knowing what you can and can't do.

Within this section, you are going to find out about what preparatory steps, and safety measures, you must be undertaking so that your exercise doesn't end up being more of a bane than a benefit.

By knowing this, you can then exercise comfortably, knowing that you have covered all the bases, and that you should have few problems, if any!

Checklist Before You Begin Exercising

Although you might be all revved up and ready to get started immediately, before you even think about beginning to exercise, or really, plan a workout program, you need to ensure that you are completely safe.

While we'll, of course, be covering some of the safety precautions that you can take to minimize your risk of anything untoward happening, the first thing that you must do is ensure that you are not in the way of the more 'general' risks.

Remember, you must absolutely go over this checklist to see if you fit into all of these categories:

1.   Do you have diabetes of any kind?

2.   Any high blood pressure problems at all?

3.   Ever had any preexisting heart conditions?

4.   Are you at risk of respiratory conditions?

5.   Do you have a medical history of premature labor?

6.   Have you tried any physical condition that has stoped you from exercising in the past?

Needless to say, most of the questions on this checklist are pretty straightforward, so you must have no trouble answering them based on prior medical check ups.

If your answer to all of these questions was a firm 'no', then congratulations, you have little or nothing to worry about, and you must be able to just follow this guide with no issues whatsoever.

However, if your answer to any of the questions in the checklist was 'yes', or if you were unsure of the answer, then it is strongly advised that you consult a doctor before you start to plan your workout program.

No, that does not mean to say that you ought to stop reading now though.

Over this guide, you will find that you are able to perform most of the recommended exercises, unless you have a specific inhibition that prevents you from doing so. Still, it wouldn't hurt if, after you know the type of prenatal exercises that you can carry out, if you get a professional medical opinion.

Better safe than sorry, right? And end of the day, you want to ensure that you are not exposing yourself to any unnecessary risk!

With this initial checklist out of way, let's move on to some of the basic safety precautions that you must be taking during your prenatal exercise.

Safety Precautions for Prenatal Exercise

Remember the golden rule that we are going to be applying in this case: Know what you can and can't do.

Really, this is the key to safe and beneficial exercise during a pregnancy, and as you are about to see, a lot of the safety precautions that you can take revolve around realizing your limits and not going long away.

As you would wait for, these limits can vary from person to other, depending on how fit they were, and how much exercise they are used to and many other factors.

Seeing as there is no formula to pursue, the truth of the matter is that no one can measure your limits better than you, thus you need to learn to do so.

1.   Do not overwork your body

Number one on our list of precautions is actually an easy and straightforward one. Whereas at normal times, overworking your body is bad, during a pregnancy, it is worse as there are too much changes within your body that need the additional energy.

Primarily, pay attention to your breathing. As you start to feel short of breath, it means that you are pushing your body a little too much.

During regular times, this can be done, but during a pregnancy, the minute you start to feel short of breath, you should scale back on whatever exercise you are doing.

Of course, there are other signs that you are overworking your body, including dizziness, nausea, fatigue, lightheadedness, and a 'chill' feeling. If you experience any of those, stop and take a break.

Should you continue to feel such symptoms, you might need to even seek medical advice.

2.   Avoid rigorous bouncing

Any sort of exercise that includes a rigorous bouncing movement is absolutely off the table during a pregnancy. Remember that when you are bouncing, your baby is going to be bouncing too, and that movement is something that you don't want to put him or her through!

3.   Avoid exercises that can cause abdominal trauma

Whereas some abdominal reinforcement exercises are fine, anything that has the potential to cause trauma to your abdomen is absolutely not. Steer clear of things that could potentially injure this delicate part of your body.

4.   Maintain a correct and proper posture

Posture is something that is extremely important during prenatal exercises, and you must always ensure that your pelvis is tilted and your back, straight.

In line with this, you should also avoid exercises that can cause you to arch your back, because coupled with the additional weight that you are carrying in your belly, this could end up causing injuries.

Exercises that bring your feet to a level that is about your hips can be detrimental.

5.   Start slowly

No matter what level of exercise you may be used to, your pregnancy has caused your circumstances to change, and you need to be willing to take that into account and gradually realize how far you can push yourself.

Start slowly, no matter how much you are used to strenuous exercise, and work your way back up!

6.   Keep cool and hydrated

The most important thing, is that you persistently ensure that you don't become overheated or dehydrated. Either of these can be detrimental to your unborn child, so you must take pains to ensure that it isn't a risk.

Avoid sport in hot or humid weather, and remember to drink lots of water at all times.

Also, wear light and breathable clothing that does not cling to your body and cause you to build up more heat than you ought to.

7.   Avoid exercises performed on your back

Generally speaking, you must avoid all of these exercises after the first trimester, but avoiding them altogether is fine too.

If you do exercise on your back, you are opening yourself up to the risk of compressing an artery due to the additional weight of your baby, and this could end up restricting some vital blood flow.

8.   Wear good shoes

Now you might not think this is important, but believe us – it is. Good exercise's shoes can provide more than comfort, and can absorb effect, provide traction, and much support.

All of these things are going to be great and helpful to ensure that your motions aren't jarring to your baby.

Based on these safety precautions, you should now have a very good idea of what you must be looking out for, and avoiding.

As you can imagine, any activity that has the potential to cause injury, like contact sports, or things such as rollerblading where you might fall, are definitely also on the 'avoid' list that you have come up with.

Equally on that list are activities at high altitudes, where the air is thinner and you will find that you will be constantly short of breath.

Equally, diving, and other related activities that could cause more pressure on your body, are also out of the question.

Basically, if you think each exercise that you are considering doing through, you must be able to now determine whether or not it is okay for you to carry it out. If in doubt, you could always consult your own medical expert.

Anyway, we are off to a pretty good start now – and it is time that we delve deeper and look at actually getting started on a workout routine!

Getting Started with Exercise

Beginning to exercise is something that can be hard for those who are not used to it. Assuming you have been exercising regularly, you may find that a lot of what follows to be things that you already know but it is worth going through this just in case there's something you missed.

Because of your existing condition, it's all the most important that you have the foundations right.

Already, you know what you should avoid, and so that must give you a fairly good grounding to start off on. However, it isn't nearly good enough if you want to have effective, beneficial, and risk-free prenatal workout routines.

Some great rules to start off any prenatal exercise are as follow:

1.   be certain to wear loose fitting and light clothes that do not restrict you or cause your body to overheat.

2.   Allow up to two hours after a meal before you start any workout.

3.   Warm up.

Yes, most of these rules are fairly self explanatory, but it is the third one that we are most interested in: The warm up.

Without a doubt, warming up is an important and highly necessary part of any exercise routine, and if you are going to be carrying out prenatal exercise, you really must ensure that your body is ready for it!

Warming Up

Basically, the goal of a warm up is easy: It limbers up your body, gets your blood flowing, and by doing so guarantee that your body is well prepared for any kind exercise you are planning to undertake.

Jumping straight in without making sure that your body is ready is a recipe for disaster.

If your muscles are tight and tense, you could end up injuring them, and if your blood isn't flowing well, then you could simply push yourself too far, too fast, and cause other complications.

Essentially, you don't wish this to happen. So the solution is easy: Warm up well!

Bearing this in mind, let's walk you through some of the basics of a good warm up, so that you are fully able to carry it out yourself, and thus getting you one step closer to having a great prenatal workout.

Remember that your warm up is, really, part of your workout itself, and it should be carried out right at the start of every exercise program!

About five to ten minutes of warming up is perfect. During that time, the bulk of it must be spent on stretching your various muscle groups. Naturally, the inclination may be to focus on the big muscle groups, and the ones that your workout is going to use most – but really, you should try to encompass as many muscles as possible.

One way to go about stretching strongly is to begin at the top and work your way down.

What this means is that you must start with your neck muscles, then go on to your shoulders, upper arms, chest, lower arms, torso, back, and waist. Various stretches could help you to stretch each of these muscles, so you must have no problem finding one that works for each, or multiple muscles at once.

After that, head lower to your groin, hamstring, upper legs, and calves as well as ankles.

As you can see, that's quite a lot of stretching, but each stretch that you perform is going to increase the benefits that you obtain. In short – you are going to be all the better for it in the long run.

When you are stretching, a common error that many people make is to stretch until they feel a slight pain. Clearly, this 'no pain, no gain' logic is wrong, and you mustn't push yourself far enough that it really hurts you.

Instead, gauge your limit, and be sure to stretch but not too much. Overstretching to the point where it is painful can really cause muscle tears.

Also, when you are stretching you must be doing so in slow and measured movements. Don't 'bounce' or 'jerk' your movement that would reverse the whole point.

For ideas of the exact stretches that you ought to be using, just refer to the many offline or online resources on the topic.

Some people tend to include a fast, slow paced cardiovascular exercise in their warm up stage, just to get the blood flowing. This is not wholly needful, but it is not harmful either, and could help bridge the difference between your warm up stage and your workout proper.

End of the day, it is largely a question of preference.

Now that we have covered the warm up and preparation for your workout, let's really sink our teeth into things, and start discussing your actual prenatal workout!

Types of Prenatal Workouts

Normal workouts come in so many different shapes and sizes, so to speak anyway.

While you may have already gathered that, due to the limitations and long list of things that you must avoid, there are severely less options that you will face – there are still quite a number that you can choose from.

Despite the limitations rule out things like, rugby and other contact sports, as well as diving, rollerblading, and anything that could result in injury, this still leaves ample other options from which you can pick what you prefer.

Roughly speaking though, if you like, you could divide the types of prenatal workouts into two main categories:

1.   Aerobic (Cardiovascular) Workouts, and

2.   Strength Building Workouts

Right here and now, we are going to be looking at both of these options individually, and letting you know what exactly you must be thinking about.

Keep in mind, there are two principal criteria for selecting the perfect exercise, and they are:

1.   Choose something that you think that you will enjoy

2.   Choose something that you think you are capable of carrying out

Put it this way, there is no point in trying to run if your sport is shot and you can hardly run for a minute before you end up gasping for breath. Also, there is not much to gain from walking on a treadmill if you find it very boring that you end up finding excuses to dodge having to work out.

End of the day, by selecting something that you like, and something that you have the ability of doing, you will be able to find the perfect prenatal workout plan!

So let's get right to it.

Aerobic (Cardiovascular) Workouts

Frankly speaking, this is the type of workout that is going to help you in many ways. Not only will it boost your blood circulation, but it'll also build your overall stamina, which will be doubly useful considering that you are carrying all that extra weight.

However, if you haven't been too active previously, you may very well have to start right at the bottom and build up your fitness. Even so, this alone is a good reason to get started sooner rather than later!

Generally speaking, aerobic exercises, or cardiovascular exercises as they're really called, help get the heart beating faster. In most cases they're used heavily by people who are trying to use weight because these kinds of exercises are a great way to spend energy.

Of course, you are not so interested about losing weight, but strengthening your cardiovascular and respiratory systems are definitely advantageous.

To get you off to a flying start, let's go over some of the options that you could choose from:

1.   Brisk Walking

Generally speaking, brisk walking just means walking at a faster-than-normal pace. Strolling in the park is nice, but it isn't exactly very strenuous, unless you really aren't fit at all.

Honestly speaking, this is one of the best types of prenatal exercises, as it is low impact, and isn't going to cause any form of 'bouncing' motion (remember, you want to avoid this at all costs).

Even within this exercise, you have numerous options. If you like, you could head over to a gym and use a treadmill, or alternatively, you could even just walk outdoors.

End of the day, the choice is yours, but remember to pick something that isn't going to turn into a chore.

2.   Jogging and Running

Naturally, jogging and running share many similar traits to brisk walking, but they are a slightly less than ideal form of prenatal workout.

In contrast to walking, jogging and running can distinctly cause 'bouncing' motion, especially if you push yourself too hard. Also, they're far more strenuous, and can really tire you out pretty fast, depending on your level of fitness.

If you have been running regularly, you could continue to do so during the first trimester or so of your pregnancy. However as you progress through it, you will want to tone things down, and maybe look to other options. Speaking of which – here's a great one…

3.   Cycling

Unlike running and jogging, cycling is definitely low-impact, and you will find that you can push yourself harder on a bicycle, or stationary bicycle, than you could by jogging or running, and still not end up having that undesirable 'bouncing' motion.

Of course, as you near term, you will find that the seat itself could become very uncomfortable, which is a downside.

4.   Swimming

Nowadays, swimming is being hailed as the best, safest, and most ideal prenatal exercise.

Why? Well, for one thing, swimming works a huge number of muscle groups at once, which means that you are going to be invariably getting a more complete workout than most other options.

Furthermore, because of the buoyancy of the water, you will actually feel 'weightless' despite the extra weight that you are carrying.

All in all, as a cardiovascular exercises, swimming actually also doubles as a strength building exercise too – to a degree. By crossing the barrier between the two in this fashion, this is really something that you ought to consider.

5.   Yoga, Tai Chi and Aerobics

Although there are vast differences between these three options, it serves to discuss them in one because they're all great forms of cardiovascular exercise that any pregnant woman can simply carry out. Also, for each of these there are several types of motions that you shouldn't do, such as anything that involves you lying on your back, or extending your legs above the level of your waist.

In short, there are risks involved with taking any of these 3 options, so you must remember that and be sure not to try to do the wrong sort of motions.

Many places nowadays have specialized prenatal aerobics and yoga classes, and you may even be able to find a good tai chi class as well. Anyway, so long as you are aware of the riskiness of certain movements, you ought to be fine.

6.   Dance

Don't laugh! While some people may not think that dance is really a legitimate form of exercise, it fills all the needs, and can give you a great workout that is fun at the same time.

Admittedly, you are not going to be able to twist your body, or leap into the air – that would be risky. But still, you can go for basic dance lessons, or just go dancing, and get a nice and fun filled workout.

In short, you could stay fit while having fun, meeting others, and just losing yourself in the music.

Did you spot anything from amongst the options that we outlined that suited your fancy? Chances are you probably did, and if so – great!

If you didn't, don't despair, there are many other types of cardiovascular exercises, such as rowing, that you could try. Honestly, to list every type of aerobic-based exercise out there would take a long time.

Suffice to say, you must be able to simply find other options, but what we have given you are some of the best prenatal aerobic exercises that you could ever find.

One other thing to consider, while we are on the subject, is the question of sports. While naturally, contact sports and anything high-impact are off the table, this still leaves a large variety of sports that you can take part in.

Such things like tennis, table tennis, badminton, squash, and many others could be worth looking into.

As long as it is safe, you should be able to do it.

Anyway, seeing as we have sufficiently covered pretty much everything you need to know about cardiovascular prenatal exercises, let's move on to the other type of exercise that we are interested in discussing…

Strength Building Workouts

Unlike cardiovascular exercises, strength building workouts aren't about just picking an activity and going for it.

Instead, strength building is all about one thing and one thing alone: Resistance training.

That means performing movements that work particular muscle groups against some degree or other of resistance. See now why swimming can help in this regard? Being surrounded by water, and moving against it, is a type of resistance training.

While any form of resistance is fine, the most common form used is simple: Weights.

By moving weights around, you are adding extra resistance to your movement, and your muscles are going to need to work harder to accomplish each and every motion. This is the foundation of strength building.

However, prenatal strength building workouts are slightly different.

For one thing, working with weights can be dangerous, especially if you are going for heavy weights that have a large amount of resistance, which are the ideal tools for maximum strength building.

Such weights however increase the risk of muscle injury, and that's something that you know you want to avoid.

Based on that, you have two options, and they are:

1.   Use lighter weights and go for more repetitions of each action, or

2.   Carry out weight-free strength building workouts

Now the first option is simple, and really doesn't need much explanation. Pick a weight that you can move simply, and then use it, as opposed to a weight that you actually have to strain hard to heft.

But it is the second option that is more attractive, because it dramatically reduces the risk of injury, while at the same time allows you to carry out a strength building workout!

Let's look slightly deeper into that option, by giving you some places where you can start pursuing it:

1.   Hamstring lifts

By lying on the right side of your body, and keeping yourself upright via your right elbow and forearm, you should then cross your left leg over your right one, in front of you.

Then, start to raise your right leg a few inches, as far as you can do so comfortably, before lowering it slowly to the floor.

Repeat the same thing for the other side.

2.   Outer thigh lift

Once again, lie on the right side of your body, but this time with your head resting on your propped up right hand. Bend your right leg if you need additional balance.

Then, raise your left leg up a little, as far as possible, and hold it there, before slowly lowering it again.

Repeat this exercise for the other side of your body.

3.   Chest muscle exercise

Clasp both your hands together in front of your chest, and press them together slowly for a few seconds.

Then, while keeping your fingers locked, pull your hands apart but don't let your grip loose. Rinse and repeat as much as you want.

4.   Squats

Stand with your feet apart, about the same distance between them as your shoulders. Then, bend your knees and lower your buttocks.

Keep your back straight throughout, and never lower yourself so that your buttocks pass your knees. Once you have reached the lowest point possible (without going too low!), slowly rise up and repeat!

5.   Wall Pushes

Stand facing any wall, with your feet apart at about a shoulder's length, and extend your palms so that they're flat on the wall. Then, lean towards the wall, bending your elbows as you do so, until your cheek is practically touching the wall (when you turn your head sidewards).

After that, straighten your body again, by 'pushing' it off the wall. Be sure to use the strength of your arms to do so.

Great, we have covered 5 weight-free exercises that can help strength building. Are there others? Certainly! But for now these should give you a firm starting point from which to work from.

Anything and everything that allows you to use your muscles against some form of resistance is going to be the kind of exercise that you are looking for, just be sure to stay away from what you know could be risky.

Equipped with the knowledge that you are, this shouldn't be too difficult.

And with that – congratulations, you are almost done finding out everything that you need to know about prenatal workouts. Let's just go over the bulk of this guide one last time, so that you can be sure that you are ready!

Starting Your Own Workouts, Today!

Armed with everything you know, you should be ready to start almost immediately, unless of course you feel that there is a need to seek some expert medical advice first.

Over the course of this guide, you should have learnt:

1.   The importance of prenatal exercise

2.   What preparation you need, and how to minimize your risks while exercising

3.   How to get started with your prenatal workout, and warm up properly

4.   All the different types of workouts that you could choose from

Does that sound about right? Be sure to check back to the appropriate section of this guide if something sounds amiss – you don't want to get caught out because you didn't grasp any part of what we have discussed.

If you are completely fine with everything you have learnt, then great! Get out there and put your body to work!

Good luck!

CHAPTER FIVE

Absolutely Everything that You Must Have For an Upcoming Baby Boy or Girl

After conceiving, going through a pregnancy, and at the end delivering your baby, you can't be blamed if you begin to think that the hard part is behind you.

Soon enough though, you will find that this easily is not the case.

No matter how prepared you imagine you are, the truth is that it is never prepared enough. There's frequently something that you forgot or easily never considered or spared a thought for.

Definitely, when you hold your baby in your arms for the first time, your thoughts are certainly not going to be on the coming months. In fact, you likely are not thinking of anything apart from how beautiful your baby is.

Are things ready for your baby when you both go home from the hospital?

Honestly, if you are a first-time parent, you may have a hard time imagining just how much needs to be ready. Up to now, you have undoubtedly been so focused on actually having a baby, that the chances are you haven't thought much past this point.

On the other hand, if you have had a baby before, then you surely have an idea of what we are talking about. But that does not make it any simple to sort things out!

Don't be afraid. This guide is here for that exact goal to help you sort out everything that you simply should have for your upcoming baby boy or girl.

Over the course of these pages, you will find you are about to discover what you should be doing, and how you should be going about doing it. We are going to explore every nook and cranny so that, when the time rolls round and you have had your baby, you are going to be fully prepared for him or her!

All you need to do is to read, understand, and then act on the advice that we will provide!

Bottom line: Your baby deserves the best, and part and parcel of that is ensuring that you have everything ready for them.

Before we delve into what exactly you need though, there's a little bit about all of this that you should know first, and a few questions that need to be answered so that you can make sure that you are on the right track…

"When Should I Start the Preparation?"

If you are asking yourself this question, congratulations, you are already thinking ahead! Many parents actually wait until their child is born, or right before, to start preparing, and this is a big, big mistake!

Here is the top advice that you can get: It's never too early to start preparation.

Once you know that you are pregnant, you already know that you are going to have a baby pretty soon, and so from that point on, you should start getting prepared.

Admittedly, as you will see soon enough, you might want to stave off some of the preparation until later on, but a lot of it can be done almost as soon as you get the results of your test of pregnancy!

By starting to prepare early, you are going to be giving yourself several advantages. First and foremost among these is the fact that you are going to have ample time to make sure that everything is sorted out.

Also, you will be able to more carefully weigh each and every decision that you have to make, so when your baby finally does arrive, everything is just perfect!

One thing that you will notice almost immediately is that there really are a lot of things that you are going to need. Some of these items may even be fairly pricey, and so you are going to have to do some financial planning as well.

Naturally, as with everything there are cheaper alternatives, and where possible, we are going to advise you on how best to proceed if you are on a budget. Also, we are going to go about this in an 'order of importance fashion'.

That means that we are going to cover the absolute essentials first, and then move on to other things that you should have too!

All things said and done, you shouldn't have to break the bank to get everything ready for your baby, but you are going to need to spend a little. Of course, if you have had a child before, or have friends whom have had children before, then you may very well find that you are able to get some of these things second-hand.

If you are scratching your head right now and wondering as to what exactly we mean don't. Let's jump straight into things and begin to look at the whole fundamentals that you ought to have on hand as soon as possible!

Absolute Essentials for a New Arrival

Of all the many things out there that you must have for your child, these are the things that, you simply can't do without!

So buckle up, and pay attention. What's about to follow are some of the most important aspects of preparing for a baby that you will ever learn about, and they're what you can't afford not to know about!

Beginning right at the top, you are about to get a full list of what you need to get ready, and some advice as to how you should go about it.

Let's get started, shall we?

Baby Diapers

Surprised that this is right at the top of our list? Well, you shouldn't be.

Truth is, baby diapers are the first things that you must get ready. They are something that you easily can't do without, and going house before you have at least a small stock of them would be catastrophic.

Imagine searching at the last minute for diapers?

Anyway, the importance of baby diapers is truly not too hard to grasp – but you can not imagine how important they are. Put it this way: A new baby can go through 8 to 12 diapers in a day alone!

Thus if you thought that you could get away with having a stock of any less than that think again. Truly, you ought to have at least a couple of days worth of diaper supply at any given time, so that you will not ever run low.

In general, there are two main types of diapers that you could use, and these are:

1.   Cloth diapers

As you can really imagine, cloth diapers are precisely what they say they are strips of cloth that are folded into diapers for babies to wear. However, cloth diapers are reusable!

That means that when a diaper is dirtied, just wash it, dry it, and you can use it again.

Also, another consideration is the fact that, being made out of different fabrics, cloth diapers tend to let children's skin 'breath', and thus prevent frequent diaper rashes, which is definitely something worth considering.

But, having to permanently be washing diapers can become a chore.

The best solution to this is that in many places (especially big cities) there are now 'diaper services', which deliver fresh diapers frequently, they also pick up the used diapers.

Of course, this is a more expensive option.

2.   Disposable diapers

Once again, the name itself pretty much sums up this type of diaper, and they are basically 'one-use' diapers that, are thrown away after dirtied.

Although disposable diapers have advanced over the years, they are still, for the extreme part, not biodegradable, and also some types can cause diaper rashes due to the materials that they are made out of.

But, it is worth noting that many brands of diaper have the advantage of absorbing more wetness than the classic cloth diapers, which can really help decrease the risk of diaper rash in some ways.

Honestly speaking though, the major advantage of disposable diapers is easily the convenience. Instead of being landed with a load of laundry, you will be able to just pick up fresh ones and throw away old ones.

Knowing the 2 types of diapers available, you must be capable to see now that there are a couple of points worth considering, and fundamentally these revolve around the fact that cloth diapers are inexpensive than disposable diapers, because they are reusable. However, disposable diapers are way more convenient.

Largely, this makes it a matter of preference. Some parents find that it is easier to start off with disposable diapers and then move on to cloth diapers later on. That way, initially at least, you won't have that much extra work with the laundry, and will be able to get used to your baby's needs!

Of course, if you are on a tight budget, you might just want to be using cloth diapers.

Keep in mind, although baby diapers are sold in 'new born' sizes, you might want to consider getting a mix of those, and a size larger.

Until your baby is actually born, it is going to be really hard to estimate his or her size, and you should definitely take into account the fact that not all babies are born at the 'newborn' size. If you have at least a few diapers around that are a size above that, you will be prepared for this possibility.

More importantly, your baby is going to grow into that larger size anyway, so it is not like you are going to be 'wasting' the diapers!

Once you have sorted out the diapers for your eventual baby, it is time we look at the next most- important thing that you should be preparing…

Sleeping Place for the Baby

Incidentally, many people think that the only option for getting a sleeping place ready for the baby is to have a crib. This isn't really true in the slightest.

Whereas it is true that a crib is a possibility, it is by no means the solely choice that you have, and you must consider your options precisely long before your baby arrives. Believe us, you will want this sorted by the time your baby does get home, so that he or she has a place to sleep right from the start.

When weighing your options you need to consider a few things, but as you will see, once again, preference is going to play a big role in your selection.

1. Cribs

As the standard sleeping place, cribs are the most common option out there. Now, many cribs have different features, like adjustable mattress heights, and some are even portable.

Foremost, the major advantage of a crib is that it will be a suitable sleeping place for babies until they are about 2 years old, and are able to crawl or climb out of the crib.

Surrounded as it is with fairly high (relatively!) fencing, your child is not going to be by accident rolling out, and will not be capable to climb out and wander around in the middle of the night without you knowing!

The moment that your baby can get out of the crib, unnecessary to say, you will have to pursue alternative options, but at 2 years old, a baby must be able to sleep in a bed even, so long as it has some form of fencing so that they cannot roll off.

Remember though that cribs can be slightly expensive, and so a good option for cheap cribs would be to either go to second-hand sales, or hand-me-downs from some friends who have had children before and they don't need their old cribs anymore.

As an added advantage, the portable versions of these cribs mean that you can have your child in whatever part of the house you are in.

2.   Co-Sleepers

Even if you don't immediately recognize the term, chances are you have seen the contraptions before.

Basically a co-sleeper looks such as a small crib that is linked to the side of a bed. Thus, as the name signifies, you could sleep with your child right beside you throughout the night.

Unnecessary to say, when your child is yet very young, this is appealing. It implies that you will have almost instantaneous access to your baby, and are able to feed him in the middle of the night without ever getting up (assuming you keep a bottle of milk handy, or breast feed).

Likewise, having your baby close by during the first months is something that many women enjoy, and it does help relax your mind, knowing that they are right there.

Regrettably, the defect of co-sleepers is that they are not as permanent a solution as cribs, because kids are able to get out of them quickly. So whereas it is a good initial option, finally you will have to seek out alternative sleeping arrangements.

If you are on a tight budget, you might want to skip this and just go for a crib, for that reason. Still, if you are able to get a hand-me-down, then that would be nice too.

A lot of the newer co-sleeper units permit for adjustable heights, and also have numerous other accessories that could help make life better, like a place to hold baby bottles, and so on.

Of course, this isn't your only option either...

3.   Bassinets

Think of a bassinet as a small bed particularly for babies. Odds are, you have encountered them before, as they are very frequently used in hospitals.

Essentially, they seems to be a 'cocoon'-like bed, big enough to just hold a child, and thus light enough to carry around. Therein lies their principal advantage, as they are greatly portable.

Instead of having to carry your child upstairs to a co-sleeper or crib each time he takes a nap, you could simply just have a bassinet that you are capable to move to whichever part of the house you are in.

By doing so, your baby will always be close by, even when sleeping.

Now, as you have probably realized, a bassinet is a great thing to have, even if you already have a crib or co-sleeper. It is portability means that you will be extending your options, and allow you a greater freedom of movement while still knowing that your baby is close enough to you.

On the disadvantage though, bassinets are just intended for child up to 3, or at very most 4, months old. After that, bassinets are in general not big enough, and even if they are, a roll could send the baby falling which is absolutely not on the cards.

For those first few months though, you will find that having a bassinet is worth it!

4.   Cradles

Despite the fact that many regard cradles as a relic of the past, the truth is that they are still as good a sleeping place for a baby as they ever were!

Additionally, you can find one very cheap, and perhaps even free as a hand-me-down or family keepsake. Cradles are frequently kept by families and passed down over the generations.

In many ways, cradles really resemble bassinets, only they tend to be lower to the ground, and are often on rockers, so that you can rock your baby comfortingly to sleep.

Still, due to these similarities, cradles also share similar advantages with bassinets, that being that they are very portable, and can simply provide you with an alternative option to your regular crib.

However, this also signifies that they share similar weaknesses, most notably the fact that after your babies is a few months old, he will perhaps outgrow the cradle, and be capable to get out of it with ease.

End of the day, just as was the case with diapers, your choice of a place to sleep for your child is ultimately just a matter of preference, as you should see now.

Again, there is the question of doubt, the very convenient option would be to have a co-sleeper and bassinet or cradle at the first time, before moving on to a crib later on.

Naturally, this option is going to be fairly costly though, especially if you are buying all of the things that you need.

So, if you are on a budget, as we have noted so far, you could either just make do with a crib alone, or rely on whatever second-hand items you are able to obtain for cheap prices (or free, of course!).

Whatever the case, be certain that you have organised at least some place to sleep for your baby before he is delivered. Leaving it till after is just going to add to the amount of tasks that you will need to perform.

Now let's move on to our next item…

First Aid Kit

Unfortunately, this is one item that every soon-to-be-parents frequently don't think about either. After all, with everything else that needs to be arranged, it actually is not the kind of thing that would pop to mind.

But it should be!

Although, hopefully, you will never ever need to use a first aid kid, the simple fact of the matter is that you probably will in some way or other. And you should be prepared for any eventuality, especially one that involves your child's well being!

Of course, you are not expected to have a replacement hospital in your own house, but ensuring that you have a properly stocked first aid kit can go a long way.

Today, you can even find kid-oriented first aid kits sold. Moreover, if you are not so certain of where you can find these, you can even make one yourself from the ground up using only a regular first aid kit.

Without any doubt, the same ingredients must be there. Plasters, bandages, iodine, and such things are actually irreplaceable. Apart from that though, you will need some other things that are very suited for children.

For example, child acetaminophen or ibuprofen would be a great place to begin. A rectal thermometer and lubricant would be another good addition.

Also, you would benefit deeply if you could find out the phone numbers of pediatricians in your area, or even emergency medical hotlines, and keep them in the first aid kit itself.

Some people even go as far as to have small 'guide cards' that detail what you could do if you are ever face to face with some of the more common problems that babies have. Either create these yourself, or see if you can find a great guide book.

End of the day, anything and everything that would help you in a medical related situation should be part of your first aid kit.

Clothing and Miscellaneous Wear

Truly, we say 'miscellaneous wear' as well because, when people say 'clothing' they actually end up leaving out a lot of clothe-related items that they mustn't.

Evidently, clothing is something that is essential. In many ways, diapers technically fall under this bracket too, but we are discussing them apart because of the sheer importance of being well stocked in terms of diapers.

However diapers aside, there are a lot of clothing that you need and you must be well stocked so that you don't have to be going to the shop or market when you get home from the hospital.

Now, we are going to go over things that you must consider:

1.   Onesies

Basically, 'onesies' are a one-piece clothing article that have an opening normally at the crotch area. Clearly, they are called an 'infant bodysuit', but 'onesies' give them nicer ring. In short, onesies are convenient.

The big advantage of onesies is that they are gender-neutral. Certainly, you may previously have had an ultrasound and know if or not you are having a boy or a girl, but if you want to begin stocking up before that, well, onesies are a good way to go.

If you live in a country that is cold, then you can use onesies as first warm layer, and then dress your kid in other clothes on top of it.

Once your baby is too young, you will not want to have to twist him into clothes. Some of the kinds of clothing may look great, but many end up being notoriously hard to dress a child in.

Thus, onesies are all the more attractive because you can slip them on and off simply.

Today, this kind of clothing come in a diversity of designs, and even styles, so you must be able to find something that looks good, but keeps the convenience and comfort of onesies.

2.   Beanie Hats

Again another good piece of babies clothing, beanie hats serve to protect your baby's head and ears, from different elements, as well as from accidentally being rubbed the wrong way when your kid tosses or turns.

So, in other words, you are not going to have to worry about your baby squirming out of his blanket, since his head will be well protected.

3.   Baby Booties and Mittens

Similarly, baby's booties and mittens equally give that 'extra mile' of protection.

Particularly, mittens are in addition useful because they will stop your baby from inadvertently scratching, and perhaps causing redness to become inflamed, or hurting his or herself.

Of course, they will also help keep your baby comfortable, and warm during cold weather.

4.   Other Clothing Items

Generally, when it comes to clothing, although we have covered the big items, there is one general rule of thumb that you simply must always follow: Opt for practicality as opposed to style.

With all the choices in baby wear that exist, there is after all going to be the temptation to dress your baby in the cutest outfit that you simply can find.

Sadly, the cutest outfit might not be the very practical, and you can find that having a group of 'cute' clothing implies that you have trouble getting your baby in and out of them when they need changing.

If you actually wish, you can, have a couple of sets of 'cute' clothing for visits to the grandparents homes, or different functions, however the majority of your baby's clothing ought to be more practical than not.

Likewise, try to avoid clothes that are too loose-fitting. Whereas it may appear to make sense to buy clothes that are a size or two larger, since your baby is going to grow. Anyway, clothes that are wery loose can be a health hazard.

End of the day, so long as you have a variety of collection of practical clothing (enough so that you don't run out!), you must be fine.

Armed with what we have listed so far, you should find that your life is a whole lot easier. Start stocking up on clothes as soon as you can, and you will find that it clears up time for you later on to spend on other preparation that needs to be done.

As far as 'must have' items for child go, clothes are absolutely on the list.

Final Words on the 'Absolute Essentials'

Over this chapter, we have so far covered the 4 'absolutely essential' items that you are going to need for your newborn child.

Now, you must notice that these are things that you can't do without. Really, if you don't sort out any one of these items, then you are going to find yourself in heaps of trouble when you get home from the hospital, baby in hand.

However, now that you know what you need to be thinking about, you are off to a great head start.

Take time to arrange what you need to purchase, what you will get from alternative sources, and what specifically you want. Already, you recognize all the choices that are in front of you, therefore making a well informed decision is the solely thing left to do.

But wait! Before you really go out and begin shopping, there are another other 'must have' items that we want to discuss.

That's right, although you currently know the absolute necessities, there are still a lot of things that you must have prepared for your baby. Even though they weren't, and aren't 'essential' enough for us to discuss them earlier, they are still needful enough for you to want to have them.

In this next section, we are going to deal with all these types of items.

For now, simply keep the urge to begin sorting out your purchases on hold for a moment, whereas you discover some other superb items that, once all is said and done, might help you to make your life a lot simple!

Much Needed Extras for a Newborn

Essentially, as the title of this section powerfully implies, these are 'extras'. Currently you would possibly be thinking that extras simply mean luxuries that you don't actually need, however think again.

Whereas it is true that you may, conceivably, manage quite well without some of these things, the reality is that they are going to end up really smoothing the path for you. Certain of the things we are about to discuss will help you to save lots of time, others can make difficult tasks a whole lot simple.

And yet others are simply downright advisable as a result of they will be of good benefit to your baby.

As a parent, anything and everything that might help your kid is naturally, too much needed! That's the underlying truth that can't be denied.

So, keeping this in mind, over this chapter we are going to be really looking at extras that will be a good advantage.

Shall we begin?

Baby Car Seats

Once you first get home from the hospital, you are perhaps not going to feel like going out for anything at all for quite some time. After all, you have your kid to take care of, which is a big demand on your time so why would you go out at all?

Well, as you will soon realize, even though your time now does have additional demands on it, sometimes you just have to go out.

What if there is an emergency, and you actually need to rush off somewhere? What if you need to pop out to the shop to fast buy something?

Really, if you have somebody else around who may look after your baby, that's fine, however what happens when you don't? At some point or other, chances are you are going to find yourself in a situation where you need to take your baby in the car with you.

And once that happens, you completely do need to have a baby car seat.

If you know any parent that has ever tried to strap their kid into a regular car seat using a safety belt, they will tell you that it is not possible. Firstly, a seat belt is not meant for someone that small, and so its diagonal strap isn't much use at all, and should even begin to rub against the kid's head, which may cause injuries.

Secondly, even if you do somehow manage to plan that dreaded strap, your baby is not going to be secure at all. Therefore you are going to find that you are going to have to try to drive whereas perpetually checking to see that your kid is okay.

In short: Don't do this!

Not solely is it dangerous, however it is reckless, and you ought to never, ever, even think about doing it.

Naturally, the solution to this current problem is easy: Get a baby car seat. Today, they are simple to find, and come in a diversity of totally different builds, and price ranges. If you look hard enough, you'll find some that are very affordable.

After you have a baby seat, make sure that it fits well and is securely fastened. At this time, you have all the liberty of movement you need... or do you?

Baby Carriers

Just as with newborn seats, these are what you will need if you plan to walk about and take your new baby with you.

Surely, if you prefer, you could easily cradle your baby in your arms as you walk, however this is going to cause your arms to ache quickly, and also it is not the secure way to carry your kid anyway, what if you by accident are knocked and drop your baby?

Keeping that in mind, baby carriers are the way to go, and they come in a large variety.

Most common are the frontal baby carriers that act as a sling in front of you wherever you can place your kid once you are walking, or even just doing household chores. Because your baby is in front of you, you will be capable to notice anything and everything about him.

Additionally, some research has shown that babies react and see a lot of things whereas they are higher up, and it will even help them to walk faster.

Anyway, having a carrier around is going to make your life miles simple, and so you must absolutely at least look around and find the options that are available.

Baby Shampoo and Washing Lotions or Soaps

As you can imagine, both of these are very necessary, however there is a small twist that you could not realize: You must be using them too! Or at least, the washing lotion or soaps.

When your baby is recently born, his or her skin is incredibly sensitive. That's why you are going to need these specialized washing lotions or soaps and shampoos. Moreover, the shampoos ought to be the varieties that aren't going to sting his or her eyes, and cause them to tear.

Not exposing your baby to the additional 'harsh' chemicals which can be found in adult soaps is critical.

Certainly, your baby's exposure to such adult soaps can also come from being in contact with you. Even if you do wash off totally, some chemicals could still remain on your skin, and might transfer over by contact, irritating your baby's skin in turn!

To avoid this, the solution is easy, simply use the same washing lotion or soap as you do for your baby.

After months, you won't need to worry about this at all, however it is a good way to dodge some of those initial issues that many parents have.

Other Miscellaneous Items

Even after everything we have discussed, there are still more things that need to be prepared, more items to be bought, and other considerations to be made. Most of these though, are really a lot more minor that what we have been discussing, and just knowing about them should suffice.

Thus, with that in mind, let's see some of the other miscellaneous items that you could want to be looking at:

1. Clean Wipes

As you can probably imagine from what we said about how many diapers you will need, you are going to have to be cleaning your baby a lot, and clean wipes go miles to help you!

2. Burp Cloths

Similarly, several babies have issues with burping, and having a burp cloth or 2, or 3, around to wipe them off can be handy.

3. Baby Bath Tub

Although many individuals use sinks until their babies are large enough for regular bath tubs, having a specialized mini baby bath tub initially can be helpful.

4. Swaddling Blankets

Basically, these are comfortable blankets that you can either wrap your kid in, or layer around the crib (or other sleeping place) for extra comfort.

5.   Diaper Backpack

If you plan to go out, you need to bring your diapers, wipes, and everything else you need along with you, thus having a diaper backpack to do so is a nice plan.

Do you get the image concerning what you must be thinking of? Certain, there are a lot of alternative items that could be added to that list, however these are by far the very important ones, and the ones that you shouldn't try to do without!

Now, you are almost done!

Now that you know what you need, there is very little left that we can offer to you, therefore with a few words, and a little recommendation and advice, we will let you go ahead and take advantage of everything that you have learnt in this chapter.

Getting Everything that Your Child Needs Ready

Knowing what you need is nice however you need to really begin taking action… now!

Believe us, there is no time such as the present, and as you will soon find, time is a luxury that no parent extremely ever has. There are, quite easy, so many things that you need to do, and you are never going to have enough time to do all of them if you wait around!

So, start right now.

Based on what you recognize, begin creating a list of the things you have, and the things you need.

From that list, try to think of where you can get the things that you need.

For example, do your parents have an ancient crib you can remove from their hands?

Mark down what you can get, and where you can get it, especially taking care to note what you are going to have to actually go out to the shops and buy for yourself.

While you are doing this, you should also start to make specific decisions regarding the various options that you know are ahead of you. Start thinking about it now, and by the time you have decided, your list should be complete.

All that remains after that is to go out there and get everything ready!

Sounds simple enough doesn't it? Well, if you move about things in the right way, and most significantly, start to do so sooner rather than later, you must have no trouble getting everything prepared in time.

Then, once you bring your baby home from the hospital, you can rest simple knowing that everything is taken care of.

Good luck!

CHAPTER SIX

Working Your Way Back to Terrific Shape after a Pregnancy

When your pregnancy is over and done with, your kid is luckily in your arms, and you are headed back home from the hospital, you will begin to understand that things have just begun.

Over the next few days, weeks, and months, you are going to progressively notice that your whole life has changed in more ways than you may ever imagine. For some, this will be a really daunting process, and it may take time for you to get used to it.

But aside from all the changes to your life totally, you beyond any doubt will want one thing to go back to being the way it was: Your body!

During your pregnancy, you'd have undoubtedly gained some weight that much is natural. Currently that it is over but, you will perhaps want to go back to being capable to fit into your favorite jeans.

Very quickly, you will find that this is easier said than done. Sure, it takes effort, however you perhaps expected that. What you may not have absolutely accounted for though is the fact that currently, with a newborn in your life, it isn't that simple to get back into shape quickly!

Don't get discouraged. Although it might not be entirely as simple as you expected, you can undoubtedly get back into terrific shape. In fact, you may find that you are even capable to be in the shape that you were before your pregnancy.

All in all, it is easily about the approach you use.

This guide is going to be your handbook to achieving the perfect weight that you want. As you leaf through these pages, you are going to find all the knowledge that you'll need to shave off those pounds, and trim your body down to the size that you desire.

More than that though, it is not simply going to be the similar old regular weight loss program that everybody is aware of. Instead, this guide is going to tailor the perfect weight loss program to the needs of a new mother – you!

In other words, everything that you simply learn from now on is going to cater specifically to the very unique desires of women who have a new baby in their life.

Right now, before we jump into the actual weight loss portion of this guide though, there are a few things that you must know to begin with. Some of these, you may already be familiar with, however it is going to be worthy going over them anyway.

Think of this as the foundation for the approach that we are going to be guiding you through.

Weight Gain and Pregnancy

Okay therefore it is safe to mention that everybody knows that it is normal to gain some weight throughout pregnancy. After all, you are carrying a total new life within your body, and so that's bound to weigh you down.

However what many individuals don't realize is that depending on a diversity of factors, you may find yourself gaining more weight, or less weight.

In general, the weight that you do gain can really be broken down into many components that add up to the whole weight, and these are:

1.   Baby – 8 pounds

2.   Placenta – 2 pounds

3.   Amniotic fluid – 2 pounds

4.   Uterus – 2 pounds

5.   Maternal breast tissue – 2 pounds

6.   Maternal blood – 4 pounds

7.   Fluid in maternal tissue – 4 pounds

8.   Maternal fat and nutrient stores – 7 pounds

As you may have noticed, all of that adds up to about 31 pounds. Keep in mind though that this is no exact figure, however for somebody who was at a healthy weight before pregnancy, the average perfect weight gain during pregnancy is about 25 to 37 pounds.

On the other hand, if you were underweight before pregnancy, you would perhaps gain 28 to 40 pounds, while if you were overweight, it would be natural to gain 15 to 25 pounds.

If you are asking yourself why all this distinction in weight gain exists, then easily think of it this way: Aside from all of the baby-related weight gain items we mentioned, the ultimate one was the maternal fat and nutrient stores.

These stores are primarily stored up energy that you and your baby can need and they are just like any other energy stores.

Soon you'll see how this links in with losing weight, but now, just remember it.

Suffice to mention, if you were overweight at first, you will want less energy stores, whereas if you were underweight, you will want more.

Another point that you ought to remove from what you have just learnt is the fact that, you actually aren't gaining that much weight at all in the long run. Most of what you do gain can, and will, be lost after you go through delivery.

What remains are mostly those energy stores that we talked about.

Of course, this is the 'perfect' scenario. Truth is, many of us really end up gaining a lot of weight during pregnancy than we 'ideally' ought to. Still, even in that scenario it is fully possible to trim off the additional weight after pregnancy!

Now that we have given you a summary on weight gain throughout pregnancy itself, let's quickly move on and tie things together with weight loss, and to do so, we need to discuss a concept that you may, or may not, already know quite a bit about…

Everything You Need To Know About Calories

Heard the term calories before? Assuming you have read anything about diets, losing weight, or something like that, you probably have at least encountered mention of it before.

Frankly speaking though, a calorie is just a measure of energy.

If that surprises you, then look at it this way: We eat food not just because it tastes good, but also because our body needs it. And while there are many components of food, such as nutrients, that are part and parcel of the reason that our body needs food, the main underlying reason that we eat is to acquire energy.

Essentially our body takes food, most notably such things as protein, carbohydrate, and fats, and turns them into energy.

So a calorie is just a certain amount of energy that can be obtained from some type of food. Look at these examples to see how that works:

1.   Fats provide 9 calories per gram

2.   Proteins provide 4 calories per gram

3.   Carbohydrates provide 4 calories per gram

4.   Alcohols provide 7 calories per gram

See what we mean now? So basically, depending on the type of food that you are eating, the amount of energy that you will be acquiring from that food could differ greatly. Some, very fatty, foods could even provide more than double the amount of energy as a food high in protein.

All this is great to know, but you may be wondering how it ties in to weight gain… and loss.

Linking Calories to Weight Gain during Pregnancy

So calories are energy, great – but why do you need to know that? What we are interested in is weight gain and weight loss; not energy.

Well, the core piece of information that you absolutely need to have to link these two things together is really something quite simple: Weight gain, in the form of fat, is caused by excess energy being 'stored' by the body.

When you eat, you are gaining energy. And when you have energy, your body uses it for a variety of functions. If however all of the energy you have gained isn't used up, then your body doesn't just throw it away – it stores it!

These 'stores of energy' take the form of fat, which is the body's way of ensuring that if you run out of energy, you have some reserves to fall back on.

That's the maternal fat and nutrient stores that we were talking about earlier. Stored energy, waiting to be used for your and your baby's needs

As a result of this, you can now reasonably be sure that on top of the weight gain caused by changes to your body itself, and your baby, the rest of the weight that you gain is going to be caused by excess energy being stored in the form of fat.

Although this realization may seem like a relatively simple one, don't underestimate its significance, because it leads us to another important concept…

Linking Calories to Weight Loss

Now we actually begin to get into the part that you are most interested in – weight loss.

Based on what you know so far, you already have stumbled upon one of the easiest ways to help along your efforts to get back shape after pregnancy, and that is: Limit your weight gain during pregnancy.

If you can keep your weight gain during pregnancy within the ideal limits, then you will undoubtedly find that your weight loss after pregnancy is going to be much, much easier!

Apart from that though, the other key realization of this section is that once your body has consumed all available energy (that it obtains from food), it burns through the energy stores (fat), changing them into energy, and consuming them.

That's why, diets are effective. In a nutshell, the way that diets work is that they scale back your calorie consumption so that you are acquiring less energy from food sources, and forcing your body to consume its reserves instead.

Similarly, exercise or anything that causes your body to use more energy, also burns through your existing energy and also forces your body to burn through its reserves.

See now how calories form a crucial foundation for any discussion of weight loss?

Knowing this, you may actually feel ready to get out there and start trimming down, and the truth is – you probably could. Understanding calories and how they work is one of the surest ways to be able to devise a plan to lose weight.

But there are other hurdles that await you when trying to lose weight after pregnancy, so it would be in your best interests to keep reading. Frankly, we are not even halfway done yet!

Firmly Resolving to Lose Weight after Pregnancy

Before you can actually start losing weight, you need to ensure that your feet are set firmly upon the path ahead of you.

Be mindful that with your changed lifestyle, it is going to take you a while to adapt and get used to all the extra demands that are now placed upon you, and this can be quite an effort to deal with on its own.

Still, that doesn't mean that you should put off getting back into shape – quite the opposite!

Truth is, the longer you put off starting to trim down and get back your former figure, it is going to get harder for you to do so. Even if you aren't putting on any extra weight, once you have somewhat 'settled' into a regular routine and gotten used to your new lifestyle, it is going to be difficult for you to change it.

Due to this, the absolute best time for you to start to try to trim down is: Right now!

In other words, you should start doing so as soon as possible, so that your weight loss efforts become part and parcel of your new lifestyle. That way, you won't need to try to fit them in after you have already settled, but will learn to cope with them along with all the other demands placed on you.

After all, what is one more demand, right?

Regardless of when you actually begin though, once you do, you need to be willing to see it through to the finish. Granted, there will be times when you find that you are forced to deviate from your schedule, and you shouldn't beat yourself up too much over this – it does happen.

But as you will soon see, there are ways in which you can minimize the risk of you having to miss a workout session.

So long as you are willing to stay the course, you will find that you will be able to attain your goals quickly, and with few problems, if any.

Of course, this doesn't mean that it is going to be a walk in the park. There will be trying times, and there will be times when you question whether or not it is worth it – but if your resolve is tough enough to know that you want to lose weight, you will get through this.

As we go through the next few sections, we are going to start giving you the best ways to start off exercising, possibly even right after you deliver your baby!

Kicking off your efforts in this fashion, you will find that you are able to get that much further, faster than you ever imagined possible.

Are you ready to begin now?

Before You Begin Any Weight Loss Effort...

Motivating yourself to succeed is all well and good, but you don't want to push yourself too far, and most importantly, you don't want to do anything that may be a risk to your health.

Considering the changes that your body and life are both going through, this is all the more important. For this reason, more than any other, you need to ensure that you are going about all efforts properly and keeping them as risk-free as possible.

With this in mind, there are a few things in particular you should know, and first and foremost, let's look at…

Warming Up and Stretching!

Soon enough, you will be starting your workouts, and when you do the one thing that you should definitely always be doing is warming up and stretching properly.

Look at your warm up as 'getting your body into gear'. Considering that you probably haven't exercised in at least nine months (or maybe longer!), this is extremely crucial because your body is undoubtedly not too accustomed to being put through strenuous workouts, or any workouts at all!

Due to that, your warm up and stretching can at least help prepare your body somewhat for what you are going to be doing.

Generally speaking, there are several options that you could choose from during your warm up. Most of them revolve around whether or not you want some form of mild aerobic exercise during it (we'll get to what exactly this is later).

That aside though, the one undeniably crucial part of any warm up is stretching, and there's no two ways about this – you must stretch!

Frankly, most people know that they have to stretch, but they don't do so because they either feel that it isn't needed, or that their body will just automatically stretch itself if they start their workout slowly and ease into things.

To a degree this is true, but when you try to just get your body to 'automatically' stretch out, you are not going to be stretching properly at all. Instead, some muscles will be semi-stretched, and others, not at all.

End of the day, getting stretched out is something that only takes five minutes or so, and by limbering up your muscles, you can avoid cramps, and worse, muscle tears!

In order to ensure that you have stretched as properly as possible, it would be best for you to devise a fixed routine, and then stick to it. Gradually, you will get used to this routine, and perform it almost automatically.

One way that works best for most people is to start at the top and work your way down.

What this means is that you should start off with your neck muscles, then work down to your shoulders, upper arms (biceps and triceps!), chest, upper back, abdomen, elbows, lower arms, wrists, waist, groin, hamstring, upper legs, knees, lower legs, and finally, ankles.

Sounds like a lot of muscles to stretch? Well, even if you aren't going to be using all of those muscles fully in your chosen workout, the fact of the matter is that they're probably going to contribute in some way, however small.

Therefore, your stretching should be as complete as possible.

Having dealt with the warm up, let's just go over something else that you should know before you start exercising, and that is…

Signs and Symptoms to Watch Out For

Whether or not you like to acknowledge it, you are in a less than ideal physical condition. Even if you were in great shape prior to pregnancy, all the changes your body has gone through over the last nine months would definitely have had some impact.

And even after delivery, those changes are going to continue to have an affect for a few weeks, or even months.

Bearing this in mind, you need to limit your risks. Pushing yourself as hard as you can is definitely off the table, and you can't train as if you are trying to make the next Olympics or something.

Even though this is true, and even if you are not pushing yourself, you should still pay attention to signs from your body that you are going too far.

Some of these signs are the kind of thing you would expect to happen when you work out, such as a shortness of breath. Nothing wrong with this, but it is a sign from your body that it has to strain itself, and you should avoid going even this far within the first few weeks after you have delivered.

More importantly however, you especially want to keep an eye open for cramps, muscle tenseness, and other 'painful' muscle symptoms.

These are more telling signs that you are certainly going a little too far, and if you find yourself facing any of these, you should stop whatever you are doing and relax for a while. Then, attempt a few stretches in the affected area, and see if the pain has calmed.

If it has, feel free to continue, but if you persistently have the same problem, you'd best contact a doctor.

All said and done, you should basically just pay attention to your body, and how it reacts to your exercise. Do that, and you should be fine.

At this point, we have covered pretty much everything you need to know before you start exercising… so all that is left now is to actually start!

Starting to Trim Down Right after Pregnancy

By now, you should be resolved as to the path before you, so all that really remains is to get started.

From what we have already discussed regarding calories, you know that there are two main ways of losing weight: Dieting to cut down on the amount of calories you consume, and exercising to burn a lot of calories than you regularly would.

Needless to say, it seems logical that the best way to proceed would be to do both!

In many ways, that is absolutely true, and we will be talking about this later. But considering you have just delivered, and you are dealing with so many new things at once, now may not be the best time to put your body through rigorous changes.

So instead of dieting and going through strenuous exercise routines, the best way to start trimming down right after your pregnancy is to approach things gradually!

Let's see how you can accomplish this…

Beginning With Slow and Easy Exercises

Were you to consult a doctor regarding when you can begin trimming down, you'd most likely be advised to wait until after your first postnatal checkup, which is normally about 6 weeks after delivery.

Although this is sound advice, because you will want to ensure that everything is fine before you start off on any heavy exercise, you could still slowly begin a few simple workouts.

Of course, despite this, you should also know and realize that you are going to be tired out quite a bit from taking care of your newborn, so don't push too difficult with any exercise that you do perform.

To start off though, you should first know that there are two types of exercises that you can choose from, and they are:

1.   Aerobic (Cardiovascular) Exercise

Mostly, aerobic is hailed as being the most contributive exercise that helps weight loss. And yes, they are also known as cardiovascular exercise, so if you hear that term being used, it means practically the same thing.

In a nutshell, aerobic exercise is any type of exercise that gets the heart pumping fast.

When this happens, you are going to be consuming more energy, and therefore burning fat faster, which is why it is so often recommended for anyone who wants to lose weight.

On top of that however, you are also going to be strengthening your heart and circulation system, because you are effectively causing more blood to course throughout your entire body.

Couple this with the fact that cardiovascular exercise is going to help with your stamina and general fitness levels, and you already have several compelling reasons to get started with this kind of workout.

So yes, any type of exercise that gets your heart rate going is good, but most commonly things such as brisk walks, running, jogging, cycling, swimming, and so on are the bread- and-butter type aerobic exercises that many opt for.

Needless to say, aerobic routines are also a form of aerobics exercise.

While most people are willing to just carry out aerobic exercises and leave it at that, there is another type of exercise out there that is worth considering…

2.   Strength Building Exercises

In contrast to aerobic exercises, strength building exercises aren't focused on causing your heart to beat faster.

Instead, these types of exercises require you to work your muscles and thus, strengthen them. To put it simply, strength building exercises generally revolve around resistance training, which consists of exercises that involve training against a resistance.

Yes, most often this means weights, though there are other forms of resistance training too.

Now you may be wondering why you have to know about this at all. After all, you are interested in losing weight, not becoming a bodybuilder – so why is this type of exercise at all relevant?

And the answer to that is simple: Strength building exercises aren't just there for you to 'bulk up'. Instead, strength building exercises can actually help you to tone your muscles so that they're firm and taut.

When this happens, you can achieve a lean and trim figure with greater ease.

Furthermore, strengthening and toning your muscles is also going to help increase your metabolism rate, because your body is going to require more energy in general.

In turn, this will help any and all efforts that you undergo to lose weight.

Knowing that both of these types of exercise have their part to play is really just the beginning, but for now, you know enough for us to leave it at that. Seeing as we have already mentioned that you are not going to want to push yourself too far, there isn't much need to go deeper than we already have just yet.

What you should realize is that both of these exercises are necessary, and you should start out, slowly, with both!

For now, until your first postnatal check up, you can ease yourself into things by doing the following:

1.   Start off with brisk walking. If you were very athletic previously, or in great shape, you could even consider short jogs.

2.   Try pelvic floor exercises, and things like abdomen crunches, to start off with.

Both of these exercise types should help you to get started on a workout that isn't too demanding. That said, you may notice that you have a small problem, and that is simply the fact that you don't have time to carry out either of these!

Admittedly, something like pelvic floor exercises, and crunches, are easier to fit in, considering you can do them from the comfort of your own home. But walking and jogging might be difficult to accommodate, which brings us to our next point of discussion.

Finding Ways to Fit in a Workout Routine

Already, we said how you must begin out your exercise routine. For now, we need to figure out how you can fit it in, amidst all the other demands on your time!

Keep one thing in mind throughout all of this: Unless you have someone to take care of your baby, you are not going to be able to leave him or her alone and go out to exercise. That much is a given.

What this signifies is that you are faced with many options:

1.   Finding someone to take care of your baby while you work out

2.   Working out at home where you can keep an eye on your child at the same time

3.   Taking your child with you when you go work out

As far as these choices go, none are very 'ideal'. Whereas finding somebody to take care of your baby when you work out look like a good option, the reality is that you perhaps will not want to leave your baby, at least not during the primary few weeks or months.

Similarly, working out at home where you can keep an eye on your baby is going to severely limit your options, and you can be sure that your workouts are going to be interrupted affairs.

As for taking your baby along with you... well, in some cases that is possible, and it is even a good option, but just as with working out at home, there will be breaks, and it could be too inconvenient.

However here is the bottom line: Of course, your baby is your prime priority. No matter what you do, and how well you plan it, your workouts come as a distinct second place (or possibly last place) when compared to your child.

So what you need to do is develop a certain amount of flexibility.

Knowing that your workouts can, and will, be interrupted affairs, you shouldn't let that get to you. Instead, snatch whatever time you can, here and there, to work out in short spurts.

When you first start out, you could use a sling to carry your child and go for a walk around your neighborhood. Some women even find that carrying out aerobic routines (with the help of many available videos, and so on) in the comfort of their own homes is an ideal solution.

Depending on what you prefer, you should find some way to fit in your workouts around your circumstances.

If you can, you should try to apply a fixed schedule to your workouts. Naturally, you are not going to be able to be too 'fixed' about it, but at least having a rough idea of when you would want to work out, all other things permitting, will help.

Establishing a routine is advantageous because once you have mentally assigned a certain time on a certain day for working out, you will slowly feel driven to work out during that time.

Initially, true, your workouts may seem to be nine parts chore, but eventually your body's reaction to working out will give you a 'good feeling' that will subconsciously make you want to work out more.

Actually, the toughest part is getting through the primary stage of working out, i.e. once your body is unused and unprepared for it. After that, it ought to be smooth sailing.

Anyway, now that we have talked about how you can fit your workouts into your postnatal routine (i.e. by being flexible about it), let's move on and look at how you can gradually move from a slow and easy workout to more strenuous activities.

And at the same time, you will also be able to incorporate other weight loss techniques, which will get you into the shape that you want to be in faster and more effectively.

So, shall we proceed?

Gradually Upping the Ante of Your Weight Loss

Earlier, we'd dealt with how, for the primary 6 weeks or so at least, until your first postnatal check up, you must go simple on your workouts.

Mind you, this doesn't signify that you ought to continue at the same level all the time. Even within the first 6 weeks itself, you will want to be progressively upping the intensity of your workouts, however taking care to warrant that you never go too far.

For this period, the rule of thumb is to take things slowly – and that signify that you must progressively up the ante, but in small increments.

However, once you have gone for your first postnatal check up, and your doctor has cleared you and given you a clean bill of health, you should be able to actually take strides forward, and go all out to get back to your former figure, or better!

It is at this point in time that the real challenge begins, and you will now be free to steadily move on to more intense workouts that will help you burn more of that surplus weight, in fewer time.

Also, seeing as you have spent about 6 weeks or so slowly building up your general fitness level, you are perfectly poised to start higher intensity workouts!

But keep in mind that although you are relatively freer, in terms of the diversity of workouts that you can now perform, you are still going to have to balance any workout you choose against the demands placed on your time by your baby.

Get used to this balancing routine – because it is something that you will be doing for a long time still, though the rewards are certainly more than worth it!

Anyway, let's look at some specific ways you can up the ante for both aerobic and strength building workouts!

Moving Forward with Aerobic Workouts

In many ways, upgrading the ante for aerobic workouts is actually the simple thing in the world: Just push yourself harder.

Assuming that up to this point you have been going for brisk walks, you might want to try jogging, or even running. Alternatively, there are innumerable aerobic exercises that you can try too.

For example, swimming and rowing, really double as force building workouts too.

End of the day, the solely rules that you need to pursue when picking how to move forward with aerobic workouts are:

1.   Pick something that you think you will enjoy doing, and

2.   Pick something that you can fit into your schedule somehow

Being a mom, in your case the preference is heavily on the second, so whereas swimming and rowing may look like good options, they will require you to actually find time aside, and also arrange for somebody to watch your baby.

Once again, it is equally possible to carry out an aerobics workout routine from home, just upping the intensity of the workout.

Choose wisely!

Moving Forward with Strength Building Exercises

Unlike aerobics, moving forward with strength building exercises is going to require that you transition from simple pelvic floor exercises and crunches on to something more: Weights.

Unfortunately, the easiest way to get started with this is to go to a gym and use the machines there. Needless to say, this may not be an option, considering you have a child to take care of at home.

So instead, you could buy some free weights and start using them to work out.

Seeing as the idea of your strength building exercises are to establish muscle tone, rather than build bulk or power, the focus of your exercises should be to perform high repetitions at low weights.

That means that you are not going to need to be hefting around heavy weights, but rather you should pick a weight that you are comfortable with, and can move easily, and then perform many repetitions of a given motion.

This is the key to gaining muscle tone, and it is what you should be shooting for.

Getting to know the different types of free weight movements that can target different muscles is something else altogether though, but thankfully you should have no problems locating more than enough resources on the matter – either through the internet, or through readily available exercise videos and DVDs.

By using free weights, you will be able to work out from home, and thus have your baby with you at all times, and retain the flexibility that you now know is so essential.

Coupling Exercise with Calorie Cutting

Last, but certainly not least, we are going to discuss cutting down on your calorie intake. If you remember, we'd mentioned that the surest and best way to lose weight was to cut down on calorie intake, while increasing the amount of calories burnt through exercise.

Previously, we weren't too concerned about calorie cutting, simply because you would need to have as much energy as possible.

Now though, you can afford to scale back on the amount of calories you are consuming, and yes, that does mean going on a 'diet' of sorts.

Unfortunately, the common misunderstanding is that to go on a diet, you need to completely starve yourself and stop eating anything that is remotely tasty. Make no mistake, this isn't the case, and in fact, starving yourself of calories and nutrients is going to be terrible for your health.

Instead, you should strive for a balanced diet that gives you sufficient calories as well as all the necessary nutrients you need to live a healthy life.

Most of us don't really have balanced diets at all, and the average American diet is generally too calorie-heavy anyway. So, you will find that simply by converting to a balanced diet, you will be cutting on calories, and embracing an overall healthier lifestyle.

If you don't know what a balanced diet is, well, you must simply be able to find information on it, or even ask your doctor when you go for your postnatal check up!

With that though, we have come to the tail end of this guide, and you are now privy to pretty much everything you need to know about getting back into shape after your pregnancy!

Getting in Shape and Staying in Shape

After hanging in with us from start to finish, you really know a lot about getting into shape. In fact, you know more than enough to actually end up in better shape that you started.

If you follow the steps we have outlined, you should have no problems acquiring whatever type of figure you have always dreamed of. By burning through the excess weight you might be carrying, and toning your muscles, you will quickly begin to see amazing results.

Throughout it all though remember that right now, as a parent; the most important thing for you to do is take care of your child.

Everything else comes second, including your efforts to get back into shape.

Still, with a little bit of effort, and all the knowledge that you now have, you should be able to do both easily!

Good luck!

www.ingramcontent.com/pod-product-compliance
Lightning Source LLC
Chambersburg PA
CBHW051256250726
48656CB00004B/1319